LOVE MUDRAS

HAND YOGA for TWO

BY SABRINA MESKO

HEALING MUDRAS
Yoga for Your Hands
Random House - Original edition

POWER MUDRAS
Yoga Hand Postures for Women
Random House - Original edition

MUDRA - GESTURES OF POWER
DVD - Sounds True

CHAKRA MUDRAS DVD set
HAND YOGA for Vitality, Creativity and Success
HAND YOGA for Concentration, Love and Longevity

HEALING MUDRAS
Yoga for Your Hands - New Edition

HEALING MUDRAS - New Edition in full color:
Healing Mudras I. ~ For Your Body
Healing Mudras II. ~ For Your Mind
Healing Mudras III. ~ For Your Soul

POWER MUDRAS
Yoga Hand Postures for Women - New Edition

MUDRA THERAPY
Hand Yoga for Pain Management and Conquering Illness

YOGA MIND
45 Meditations for Inner Peace, Prosperity and Protection

MUDRAS FOR ASTROLOGICAL SIGNS
Volumes I. ~ XII.

MUDRAS FOR ARIES, TAURUS, GEMINI, CANCER, LEO, VIRGO, LIBRA, SCORPIO, SAGITTARIUS, CAPRICORN, AQUARIUS, PISCES
12 Book Series

LOVE MUDRAS
Hand Yoga for Two

MUDRAS AND CRYSTALS
The Alchemy of Energy protection

LOVE MUDRAS

HAND YOGA for TWO

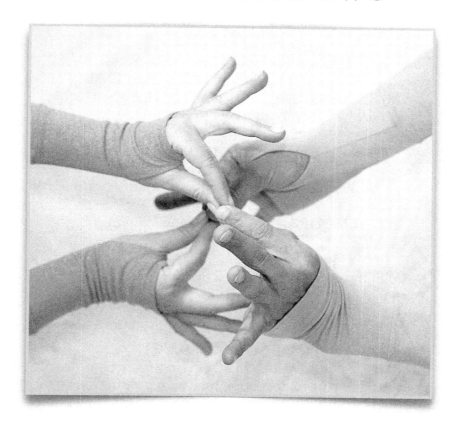

Sabrina Mesko Ph.D.H.

A MUDRA Hands™ Book
Published by Mudra Hands Publishing

Cover photo by Holly N. Hughes
Chapter Title Photography by Ken Pivak
Mudra Sets & Close-ups Photos by Holly N. Hughes
Symbol Design Kiar Mesko

On the cover Mudra for Tranquilizing your Mind

Printed in the United States of America

First MUDRA Hands Publishing Edition
December 2017

Manufactured in the United States of America

ISBN-13: 978-0692045305

ISBN-10: 0692045309

The greatest Gift in Life is to Love

and to be Loved in Return...

CONTENTS

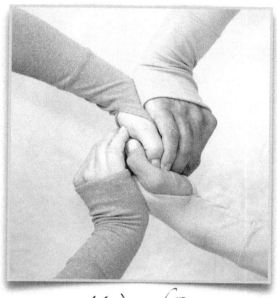

Mudra of Joy

INTRODUCTION

The moment you touch your lover's hand for the first time, a galactic shift occurs. Your energies intertwine and you merge on invisible realms. Mudras are the navigation system to help you navigate this beautiful journey of communication and love between the two of you. And this book is your map to the heavenly realms of unconditional, everlasting love.

I always knew I wanted to "save the world", and guess what? Mudras can actually do just that - they can help you save yourself and in this case save and elevate your relationship. As I look at my extensive work with Mudras that spans thru a few decades of numerous books on this fascinating topic, I still marvel at the incredibly powerful and transformative effects this ancient technique offers to all who delve into it. Mudras truly are an everlasting treasure and the more our world becomes dependent on outside "gadgets" and we are encouraged to succumb and allow them to run our life, the more I remain a firm believer that we possess all tools for self improvement, self-realization and everlasting love within ourselves, or more precisely - in our own hands and hearts.

Our continuous search for answers outside of ourselves eventually brings us back to that sobering moment in front of a mirror, when we are forced to look upon the reflection of who we are, who we've become, and what we surround ourselves with. We allow life to take us places without our conscious awareness, until suddenly one day we wake up and hopefully recognize the power within us - to lead a life with our mindful participation, a life where we actually consciously create our dreams and pursue our wishes and desires. Mudras ignite this self realization process and propel you into stratosphere of higher consciousness. And while they occupy a very special place in my heart, there is another topic that I feel compelled to include in my work - the magnificent and majestic power of love.

Each and every human being in this world needs, deserves and desires to be loved. Conscious projection of love towards anyone can alter and improve their overall state. I used to conduct this "experiment" throughout my life, sometimes in most challenging circumstances. When someone was unkind to me, I consciously sent them a powerful ray of unlimited love and within minutes their disposition changed drastically.

Of course not every challenging situation can be resolved so easily. But it is indisputable that love is a force of tremendous magnitude, beyond our ability to understand its grandeur and absoluteness. Throughout our lives each one of us has various experiences of love as well as heartbreak, and hopefully the blessing of being loved in return. Yes, you may love someone, but if they do not love you back, you are only half way there.

Love and relationships are an ever important human preoccupation, for it is what matters most in our lives. And it is precisely here that Mudras can play a very crucial role when seeking deeper experiences of love between two partners. Because Mudras raise your consciousness and help you remember your true soul power, they are incredibly effective when practiced together with someone you love.

When your fingers touch, something truly short of miraculous happens. The healing aspect is obvious, but there is something else. It is like a sacred gateway that only the two of you feel has opened, and Mudras are the invisible and mysterious key. In the hidden world of interconnected energy fields that the two of you enter, you will find the delicate yin yang balance while energetically aligning yourself with your partner in order to heal, purify, embellish, and ascend the experience of love. The practice of majestic and transformative Mudras will take you both into the land of faraway places where unconditional love is the rule, and your hearts can open without hesitation or fear. After your Mudra practice, when you are both in a higher state of consciousness and your hearts are optimally open to give as well as receive, you are able to utter unconditionally loving, accepting and affectionate words for each other. This devoted verbal exchange between two people, void of all negative aspects but clear in resonance and pure in its purpose, has the power to heal, and further elevate your relationship into a state of blissful unity beyond your dreams.

My wish and the mission of this book in your hands is to present to you the indestructible power achieved when using healing Mudras for the exalted principles of communication within a love relationship. With dedicated Mudra practice, the two of you are granted entry into the sacred chamber of true unconditional love. Allow this intricate guidebook to show you the way so that you too may benefit from this formidable ancient technique.

If you practice Mudras on your own, you know and understand the positive impact they offer and the immense changes they create in your life. You understand the way your energy field instantaneously opens up and expands, eliminating all obstacles while magnifying your power. But practicing Mudras with a partner takes everything to a different level. Let me put it this way; imagine taking a walk on a beautiful endless sun-kissed beach or flying weightless thru mesmerizing galaxies. And while the first option has its joys and magical moments, the second changes your life in an irreversible way. There are forces at hand - literally - that transport you into a whole new world of joint higher frequency, and that my dear reader, brings you terribly close to home, your true original home of Universal Unconditional Love from which all life begins and returns to.
Now, you're on your way...

This book is meant for all couples of this world since Mudras and Love both have one strong common ground - they are Universal. May this evolving journey, bring you and your Mudra - mate a most profound and everlasting state of joy and bliss, so that together, you may conquer the world.
Endless Blessings,

Sabrina

Part One

Instructions for Practice

Just because Mudras seem simple it does not mean that they are passive or forceless.
In fact they are the precisely opposite.
They ignite invisible powers with such intensity that your life is transformed.
Combining them with the power of love between you, you enter a new world, beyond touch, sight or sound.
It is a finer, subtler, exquisitely invisible world of mysterious other dimensions,
that are only revealed to souls before entering or after departing this world.
The instructions for activating this sacred blueprint must be carried out
with utmost dedication, lear intention, and acute precision.
Only then can you enter the sacred pyramid of this ancient knowledge
and participate in this marvelous master plan.
And remember, upon entering, your life and your love relationship will never be the same again.
Trust, that everything is happening at the precisely perfect time for you both.
And the time is now.

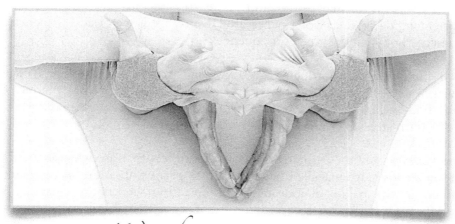

Mudra of Receiving Empowerment

WHAT ARE MUDRAS?

Mudras are ancient healing hand gestures and yoga postures where you are using various intricate positions of fingers, hands, and arms. These beautiful gestures originated in Egypt, over 5000 years ago and were used by high priests and priestesses in sacred healing rituals. Mudras can be found in every culture on earth and are truly universal. Mudras are clear, simple, yet inexplicably powerful tools for exalted communication between two partners. They are like fine tuned formulas to repair, redirect, and reconfigure your energy patterns of interaction.

HOW DO MUDRAS WORK?

Mudras are quite powerful, highly effective, and offer immediate healing effects. They are very easy to do, and can be practiced by anyone who can move their arms and hands. Simply by joining your fingertips in specific combinations, you are directly affecting your entire physical, emotional, mental and subtle energy bodies, opening and reactivating your energy currents and chakra centers.

Mudras have to be practiced with proper breathing techniques to help facilitate and expedite the healing process. They are excellent for unblocking congested energy clusters within your subtle body that may be preventing healthy functioning, and are thus diminishing chances for disease.

BENEFITS OF YOUR MUDRA PRACTICE

Emotional and mental states continuously transform and shape your energy body, in response to environments, other people and events that occur in your life. You may have a mentally challenging day, which won't necessarily display in your physical presence, however your subtle energy body will feel the consequences.

Likewise, you could be going through an emotionally stressful situation, which again won't show in your physical stature, but will affect your energy body. If these dynamics continue, your physical body will eventually suffer and display unharmonious manifestations as a result of long - term stressors on finer energy levels.

Mudras work on precisely these finer, subtler energy levels that are invisible to the human eye. Numerous energy current called nadis end in fingertips, in addition to smaller chakra centers that are in the palms of our hands. Connecting the energy currents from two opposite poles - meaning the right and left side of your body while you are practicing a Mudra, creates an energy surge, opening up blocked nadis and increasing vital energy flow for regeneration and vitality.

CHAKRAS, NADIS AND MUDRAS

In your body, along your spine, there are seven major energy centers, called chakras that are spinning in a clockwise direction. These vortexes of energy affect every aspect of each specific region where they are, and play a decisive role in your general state of physical health as well as mental and emotional disposition. In addition, there are 72.000 energy currents called nadis, running through your body, like subtle energy "veins", intricately interwoven and part of your complex and highly sophisticated energy body field.

Your energy body is like an invisible sensory engine that is quite sensitive and quickly responds to outside stimuli like environment, sound, food, aromas, color, and certainly people. When it comes to interaction between two partners that are connected with emotions of love, Mudras help to balance, harmonize and magnify these delicate states, while evoking your ability to actually sense the subtle energy interaction, merging, and the tremendously powerful energetic bonding. The invisible individual frequencies of two partners that are energetically connected must be somewhat compatible in order for them to experience the emotions of love and attraction for one another.

The fact that these two people resonate on a very similar or same frequency level, creates a substantial magnetic effect on both sides, thus expanding and crystalizing their joint power making it tangible even to an outside observer. The magnetic force creates an actual energy "pull' towards each other, which can be difficult to resist, regardless of circumstances.

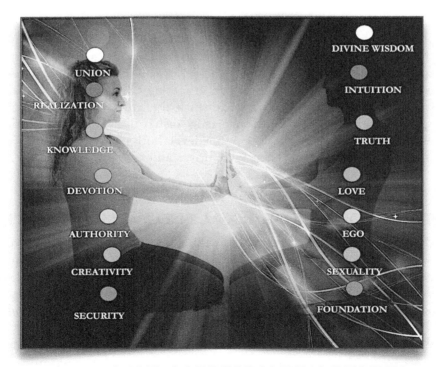

CHAKRAS AND CORRESPONDING DESIRES

How do Mudras for Two work?

The disciplined practice of Mudras ascends the magnificent yet invisible energy interaction to a whole other subtle level of immense strength, magnetism and produces a combined energy current that has a very transformative effect on the two practitioners as well as those who simply observe this interaction.

Once we understand how intricate the energy system and Mudra combination is, imagine you multiply that with endless options when you connect these two compatible practitioners. Now you are combining two tremendous sources of raw life force, joining them consciously and with awareness.

Your focused and centered intention with each combined Mudra, creates an invisible surge of energy that affects both practitioners in a most beneficial and transformative way. A simple placement of interlacing your hands and fingers creates an instant energy bind between two hand chakras as well as interlaced fingers, thousands of nadis and this seemingly harmless position exudes a potent flare of combined force. You both feel charged, stronger, and coordinated for you are merged deeper than it appears. What is happening that is invisible to the human eye?
The answer is quite fascinating.

Aligning your Subtle Energy Bodies

When the emotions between two people are loving, and they sense a mutual attraction, there seems to be a hidden force that is pulling them together and no matter how near or far they are, they can sense each other, sometimes think of each other at the same time and almost communicate on some kind of untouchable level. What is happening is that their individual frequencies are "sensing" each other, attracting each other, and finally unifying in perfect resonance. When outside influences disturb, deplete or distract this perfect unity, the two beings feel the shift and experience it as disharmony, discontent and conflict. When this joined frequency vibrates at its optimal level, both partners feel exalted, content, and full of vital energy yet peaceful. Their love thrives and ascends.

Mudras ~Tools for Exalted Communication

We are incredibly sensitive; yet we forget about this fact, and do not properly tend to this fine energy element of our existence. In an intimate relationship everything is magnified in a positive sense and possibly also in negative, weakened state. Therefore it is essential that you and your partner are aware of these fine delicate dynamics between the two of you, and consciously nurture and dedicate loving energy to cultivate and protect this beautiful energy field between you. Mudras are beyond ideal for this specific purpose since they offer you easy, fast and supremely powerful tools to keep your love harmonious and invigorated.

They help you purify, magnify and exalt this precious connection so that you both truly experience blissful union of two souls. Whatever Mudras you select, be aware that the energy between you two will soar and create an immense jolt of energy rocketing you into spiritual awareness and mutual activation of your higher consciousness.

What happens next is that your relationship changes. It ascends into spheres you never dreamed possible, your attunement to each other becomes so natural and flowing, that you understand and tangibly feel what an unconditional, loving and harmonious resonance is and the magnitude of its power.

You will achieve the desired state of inner peace, astonishing focus and concentration, supreme health and mastery of your mind. This is the absolute best possible position for you and your loving partner to enjoy a most fulfilling love relationship. Everything you need is at your fingertips, for you can practice Mudras anywhere; all you need is time, dedication and your love. Leave the rest to Mudras and let the magic begin.

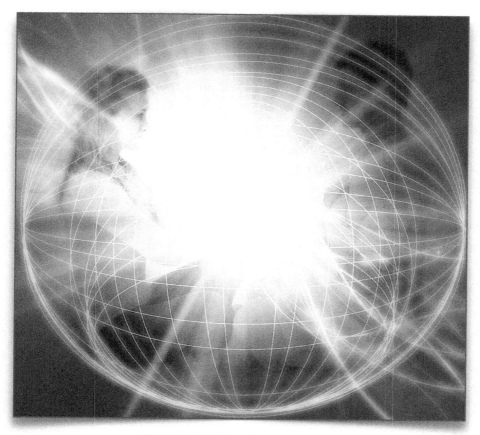

SHARED ENERGY FIELD

YOUR HANDS AND THE COSMOS

In addition to revitalizing your entire energy body, Mudras offer an impressive benefit to fine tune your mental abilities, balance your emotional states and uplift your spiritual states. This specific effect occurs when selected fingers are joined, or kept apart, as well as palms turned in various directions, or details of each posture in relation to your body.

Mudras are not isolated gestures, disconnected from your physical posture or placement as far as height in relation to your body, and direction of the pointed fingers. Every singular detail does matter and precision is of utmost importance, especially when your aim is to eliminate a challenging mental obstacle or increase a desired ability, improve a weakened state, as well as develop special gifts.

Here the fascinating relationship between the solar system and your hands comes into play. The right side of the body is ruled by the sun, the male and mental aspect, and the left side is under the influence of the moon, feminine, emotional energy. Furthermore, each finger relates to a specific planet, creating intricate network of interconnected triggers in your disposition, strengths, weaknesses, challenges as well as special abilities and gifts. This is one of the reasons why it is actually of great importance which fingers do connect and which hand is on top of the other, as well as where they are held in relation to your body.

Thumb - God - Mars - willpower, logic, ego
Index - Jupiter - knowledge, wisdom, self confidence
Middle finger - Saturn - patience, emotional control, challenges to overcome
Ring finger - Sun - vitality, life energy, health, love
Little finger - Mercury - communication, creativity, beauty

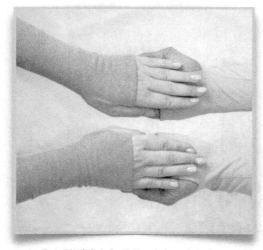

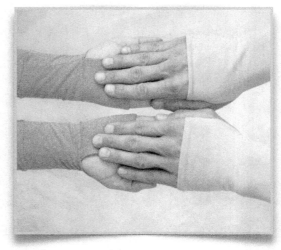

SAFETY & PROTECTION   COMFORT & TENDERNESS

HEALING BREATH WITH YOUR PARTNER

The next important aspect is your breath. Breath has immediate connection to your emotional state, whatever that may be. Just think how you breathe when you are tired, stressed, less enthusiastic or when you are excited, happy and peaceful. When practicing controlled breathing you will immediately calm and center your entire being.

This truly is a very powerful dynamic, but when you are practicing synchronized breath with your partner, the power created is tangible. It is actually one of the essential needed steps when practicing Mudras together. Usually your breath automatically synchronizes with someone that is close to you, because as does sound work in a fascinating concept of resonance, so does breath. What does that mean? When one of you has a strong, calm, confident breathing pattern, the other weaker, restless, and unfocused partner will eventually begin to resonate with the breathing tempo and pattern of the stronger, calmer partner.

The breath should always be thru the nose and centered at the solar plexus stomach area, expanding when inhaling and contracting with each exhalation. Usually Mudras are practiced in a slow, long deep breathing rhythm. Occasionally when so noted, you may use the fast, short breath of fire, which works under the same principles, but at a faster pace. Always use your own judgment to remain comfortable during your Mudra practice and if needed, return back to the long, deep breathing to complete a three-minute Mudra exercise.

Looking at the breath component from a more esoteric perspective, when you harmonize your breath with your partner's, you enter a state of deep visceral coordination that expands your consciousness and propels you into understanding the vastness of all existence. Everything alive needs to breathe and this is the law of life. Breathing in unison not only creates an instant state of calmness and connectivity with your partner, but it submerges you into a state of cellular coordination. Your physical bodies unify in an existentially raw concept and this adds an element of profound energetic fusion. Remember, your breath is the voice of your soul.

POSTURE

The posture is extremely important, so that you allow all your energy centers to open up, function at their best capacity for equal and harmonious exchange and energetic connection with your partner. Sit comfortably, the shoulders remain down and relaxed, back straight with a nice long neck.

EYE GAZING

While we usually close our eyes during meditation, it is an entirely different experience during *Mudra practice for Two*, because your eyes remain open and play an intricate role in this technique. While you can close your eyes during meditation and experience your inner vision, now you can choose to do something even more beautiful than that.

You can look into your partner's eyes, gaze into them for minutes without uttering a single word. Everything you need to communicate with them is in the eyes, for they reveal the deepest essence of one's soul. Remember, when you first met, you looked at each other's eyes deeply, openly, they took your breath away, mesmerized you and instantaneously eliminated all sound. It was just the two of you and your melting in each other's gaze. It was that magical moment when you knew your life changed and your heart skipped, your breath disappeared and all you could see were the eyes. And now you still look at each other's eyes but you do not savor the moment, you do not make the time, stand still and decide that this is precisely what you wish to be doing for the next ten minutes. Just looking at the one you love, without conversation, needs, comments, storytelling or questions. No, just be.

And you may laugh, you may sigh and then you most certainly will cry. For you will remember how it was when you first saw these eyes and how beautiful the world seemed at once. And how you could go on every day living with this luxury of having these eyes right next to you, yet you perhaps forget and waste your precious time by starring at something much lees vibrant and lovely. Every second you have, where you could again recall that moment in time and grasp that precious connection that happens with the eyes, every such instant should be enjoyed and soaked up, for it is a passing one. Mudras will not only take you back to that time when you remembered and "recognized" each other's Soul, but they will do much more. They will take you further into the future, deeper into your heart, and eventually pull you into an entirely different existence as a couple. Suddenly, you will lose the limited identity of being one and you will become two, merged into one. You'll cease to feel divided, and experience the true unity of two souls.

MEDITATION

To learn how to experience inner stillness, you can practice this simple Mudra for Developing Meditation. Sit with a straight back and face your partner, knees touching lightly. Lift the hands up to the solar plexus level and with the four fingers of your right hand together in a straight line, feel the pulse on your left wrist. Press lightly so you can feel your pulse in each fingertip. With each beat of the pulse inhale, hold, exhale and again hold for equal counts. This will help you enter a state of deep relaxation and will guide you towards experiencing the beginning of a meditative state. Look deeply into each other's eyes and be conscious of the oneness with your partner and all Universe. Project unconditional love and unity while gazing at each other. Practice for three minutes. **Breathe long, deep and slow.**

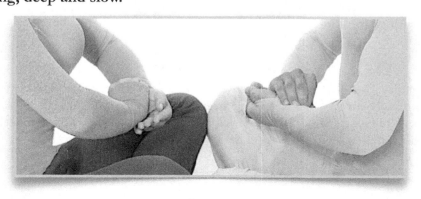

AFFIRMATIONS

During the Mudra practice your mind becomes still and open to positive input. This is an excellent time to consciously establish positive inner dialogue, and reaffirm an affirmation that you both selected. You may say the affirmation out loud before or after Mudra practice, or you may repeat it in your mind during the entire exercise. You will project the desired outcome and utilize the tremendous power of your collective minds to help bring you closer to fulfilling your goals and dreams. Affirmations are always practiced with an open perception that allows the Universe to bring about your wish, while you do everything you can to help this become a reality. However, once you have done your part, allow the Universe to manifest it in whatever way is best for you and the higher good of all.

YOUR PRACTICE SPACE AND TIME

The ideal space for your practice should be quiet and peaceful; however, once you advance in your practice you will be able to connect instantly with each other even in challenging, stressful and less peaceful circumstances. For example: if you are facing a difficult immediate situation, the practice of Mudra together will instantaneously bond you, reconnect you, and empower you, so that you may regain your inner balance, and find fast solutions to increase your joint strength when overcoming the challenge. This is very essential and most valuable.

YOUR TIME COMMITMENT TO PRACTICE

To establish a regular practice time, set aside a time where you are both not rushed, and can dedicate at least ten minutes to each other without interruptions or distractions. If this is a challenge, start with a short amount of time - five minutes. Each Mudra needs to be practiced at least three minutes. Allow two additional minutes for sitting in stillness. As little as this may seem, do not underestimate the power of Mudras. When you develop a regular practice schedule, you will feel the positive effects faster and stronger, and may lose yourself in Mudras and each other for an hour at a time.

YOUR REWARDS

When you add to this potent *Mudra practice for Two* a clear and light-bearing mission, you have a force of tremendous potential with the ability to change, uplift, inspire and transform anyone who is seeking answers, knowledge and purpose. By practicing Mudras with your partner, you will transcend your challenges and eliminate any friction, conflict that you are facing, and establish a new harmonious and compatible energy current that will embellish the natural connection which originally brought you together, so that you may finally ascend into the highest realms of experiencing the true meaning of unconditional love.

Your Conversation after Mudra Practice

In "Speak from Your Heart" sections you will find laid out a most authentic example of unconditionally loving conversation that you can develop with your partner. After your Mudra practice, you may sit in silence and enjoy each other's synchronized essence of profound mutual love and adoration. Or you may choose to share your love with words for each other, infused with wisdom and kindness of your immeasurable love. Words are most powerful and while sometimes we may allow them to get clouded with ego and carelessly escape and hurt the other, they do have a tremendous power to heal, elevate and transform your relationship into higher spheres where you truly become untouchable.

After Mudra practice you will find it much easier to communicate in a loving, kind, tender, and honest way. All fears and unnecessary emotions that may have blocked your spoken communication will fall away and you will return to your essence – the love between you two. Words from the heart are like a meteor shower upon you…soothing, majestic, and full of magnificent blessings for one another. They help you remember who you truly are - two angelic beings in human form, breathing as one and sharing your light with the world. The world needs you, we all need you, let your glorious light shine with the purity of your love.

What happens during Mudra Practice?

In any relationship, communication is of utmost importance and it is often a challenge to find the balance between enough interaction or attention for the more communicative partner, without seeming to be too needy for the more quiet, reserved one. Mudras are truly a gift in this aspect. Why?

Because during Mudra practice, you feel a profound connection with your partner, you have their time and attention but it is not too demanding for them, because no conversation is needed. Mudras offer the luxury of "speechless conversation" which is so much more powerful than one can imagine. You simply have to experience it yourself. Everything you desire from a partner in regards to communication is given to you; their presence, attention, warmth, tenderness, gentleness and most of all the tremendous wave of your love for one another that envelops you and sends you into a blissful state beyond description.

But of course it is the exquisite combination of the two of you that creates that energy bubble, impenetrable to outside forces and magnified with such potency that you become invincible. Mudras will calm your sensitive female nature, soothe any restlessness of your male dominiering side, transcend any energy imbalances you have within your relationship, and help you discover first the divinity in each other, and then you together, as an extraordinary energetic entity in all its majestic beauty and power. No matter how strong or independent you are, your heart still needs a partner in order to experience this kind of ultimate manifestation of unconditional love.Mudras will transport you to your secret place of higher love that you always longed to know. Now it is here. Enjoy and cherish each precious moment together, for you are fortunate beyond words.

Part Two

About Love

When you fall in love for the first time, you feel like you understand everything about life, but you don't.

When you lose your love, you feel like life is over, but it isn't.

When you search for love, you feel hopeless, but you are not.

When you get wounded in love, you feel you will never recover, but you will.

When you learn to love yourself, you are taking the right step, and you know it.

When you meet your soul mate or twin flame, you become alive, and you feel it.

When you love unconditionally, you understand you will never lose him, and you won't.

He and you are bound forever into eternity, beyond space and time.

Love him and thank him every day that he found you, for love IS everything that matters.

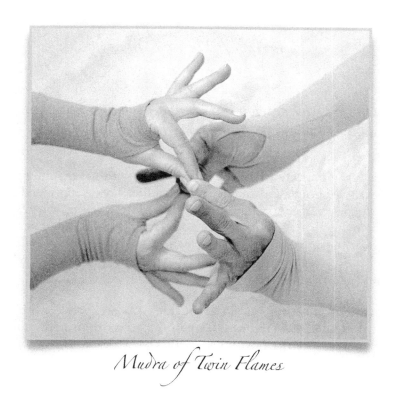

Mudra of Twin Flames

The Two Principles

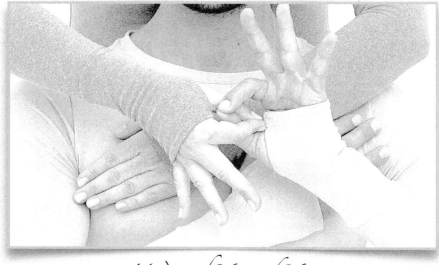

Mudra of Yin and Yang

Love Mudras will help you develop a deep and profound understanding of your Soul's Yin and Yang essences, so that together you may balance your power.

As humans we have the expected tendency to identify with a very limited belief about who we are and what we should and can expect from life. This is ingrained in us since our first breath and shapes our entire life from that moment on, whatever the family environment is, the dynamics, the culture, religious observations and general expectations of what we should or must accomplish in our lives. The scope of expectations to fulfill is truly limitless and unless we are born with the heart of a seeker, we will most likely succumb and try to fit in the mold as best we can.

However, chances are your nature is different and you are precisely this seeker, who strives to find out more, has the strength to open the secret door and courageously walk through the dark hallway until the next secret door reveals itself. You want to understand the depths of your Soul and the deepest compartments of your heart. In this inner search you will meet with two distinct energies, the male and the female within you.

This very unique combination that lives inside your core is truly your Spiritual imprint from all your combined lives of your far past. If you experienced the majority of lives as male you will certainly feel more comfortable with that specific energy. And likewise, if you lived more lives as a female, your familiarity with these aspects will be more dominant.

I love being a woman, even though I do have very strong definite male principles within my personality. I believe it is most important to understand these intricate elements within yourself and be lovingly comfortable in your own skin. Not trying to fit a mold, but just finding your own inner balance where your Soul energy can truly thrive and express itself most freely. We all have a male and a female side within us regardless of the sexual definition of our physical body or our sexual orientation. It is absolutely absurd to imagine all women are entirely feminine and all men are nothing but masculine in every aspect of their lives. Each one of us is an absolutely unique combination of these aspects and this intricately intertwines with our general personality, gifts, desires, life pursuits and certainly love relationships. These two distinctly different energies do not make you less of a woman in case of your male strength, or less of a man in case of your deeper understanding of the feminine manifestation; in fact the dynamic expands your understanding of these two formidable forces.

The key as always is finding your balance within, no matter what unique combination you posses. And furthermore, when attracting and merging with your ideal partner, your awareness of who you are and how you relate to these two forces will play an intricate part in every aspect of your relationship. Ideally your partner and their specific combination should embellish your strengths and positive qualities, while you offer them an equal boost of energy in return. The ideal combination for yourself and your partner will allow you to find an absolute balance within your male and female energy levels so that together you are unified in harmony and peace, not fighting each other but embellishing and strengthening each other. Again, this goes for whatever body you are born with or whatever sex your partner is.

Your partner and you are bound by energies much more complex than just the basic physical attraction. The perfect balance of these two energies creates a very special embellished bond that makes the two of you invincible and propels you towards the optimal state of existence in human form, meaning a perfectly balanced two individuals that create a complete oneness of two beings. The fact that we are all interconnected, for we are all from the same source comes into realization for it is only by balancing these two forces that you have a chance of rising to this possible ascended level of Higher Consciousness and existence.

Perhaps that is the reason we are always in search of our other absolute half - because without the other half, we can not rise above the limitations of this dimension. Whatever combination this pairing manifests in, it is your destined journey to your true home. The secret formula is not something you can find outside of the relationship, the secret formula is in fact inside the two of you - together.

Understanding & Knowing Yourself

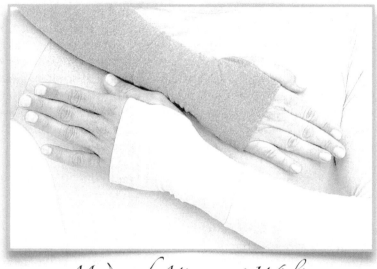

Mudra of Attunement Within

Love Mudras will help you discover your truth, your dreams,
fantasies and wishes, so that together you may manifest them precisely so.

Have you ever observed and understood all intricate elements of your personality?
Have you embarked on a self discovering journey and tried to unravel the mysteries of you?
Why you are the way you are, your belief system, your disposition towards life, but most of all your relationship with yourself? Do you understand and most importantly, do you love yourself? This would entail some deep soul searching and honest self-observing.

Imagine seeing yourself as someone else is seeing you. Are you capable of doing that? For a moment, step out of your limited "bubble" of existence and truly expand your ability to observe yourself from a completely neutral perspective. Knowing yourself is not an easy task. However, let us say this, not knowing yourself and living with yourself sure is a mighty challenge. It means you can not trust yourself because you actually do not know how you will behave, what you will do, and mostly how you will feel under unexpected given circumstances. And if you don't trust yourself, you certainly can't trust others.

How do you get to know yourself? Stop with the constant business of your restless body, untamed mind and wildly running emotions, and become completely still and centered. Just breathe and give yourself a space of absolute silence and peace.

Now, begin an inner conversation with a kind loving demeanor and inquire within. Ask yourself how you feel at this particular moment. Next, examine why you feel that way. Finally, patiently ask yourself what you want. Know that you will never get what you want if you do not know what that is. And in worst case scenario, you may receive what you want, but if you can't recognize it, you will most certainly also lose it. But, you will receive what you desire, if you know what that is.

Loving yourself is the last step in this preparation process. If each and every day your inner dialogue begins with a scolding attitude, you cannot possibly expect a cheerful, optimistic and successful day, for you carry within yourself the worst critic of all times - you. If this critic is allowed to rampage thru your life, you will continuously walk around with a beaten, pessimistic and weak disposition, full of self doubt and insecurities. Quite often, being different will cause you to question your own self-worth and face more critical challenges from others.

If you are unlike everyone else around you, chances are you will be sticking out of the crowd and possibly bothering some, for you may not fit into any typical category. That was always my case throughout my life, however I am of a very curious nature and wanted to understand and know myself clearly and without hesitation. It was not difficult to see and understand all my imperfections, but it was certainly less fun accepting them.

The most challenging aspect was to take time and effort to be kind and loving towards myself, for my nature is to help others in a most dedicated way. Forgetting myself during the process always provided lessons to learn, so that I was forced to put myself into the equation and develop space, time and love towards myself as well. I am still working on that and most likely will for the rest of my life. It is only under these conditions and once this aspect of yourself is understood in a most profound way, that one can lead a healthy and happy life, and attract a similarly complete person into their closest energy space. By consciously and with awareness changing your inner dialogue while transforming the merciless inner critic into the kindest, most encouraging, accepting, and loving friendly supporter, you will become your own best friend. This is the absolutely non-negotiable first step towards a healthy relationship. Become your own best friend and now you can begin to attract others who will likewise become your best friends. A most equal and loving relationship must be based on a strong, unwavering and loyal friendship, filled with absolute trust and unconditional support.

This way you are building your house of love properly and with a base that will sustain all earthquakes of life and floods of challenges. You will be able to remain standing thru the wildest of hurricanes and storms, always providing a safe haven for yourself and your loved one.

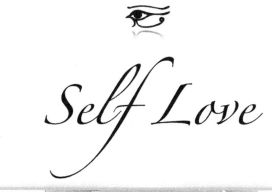

Self Love

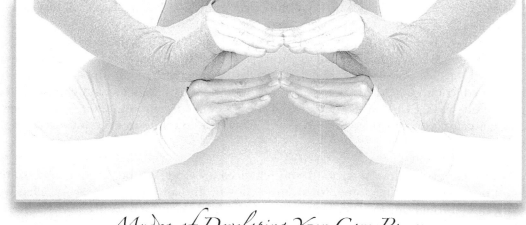

Mudra of Developing Your Core Power

Love Mudras will help you find the essential source of love within,
so that together you may build your indestructible Temple of Love.

You may dream of and visualize the most fantastic loving partner, but the simple unavoidable fact is, that unless you love yourself, you cannot even begin to expect this dream to come true. The self-love begins with your body and since that is truly a challenge with all the unrealistic "role models" out there, you may experience some harsh self-criticism. But just think; how can you expect someone else to love, worship and adore you if you don't? That's simply impossible.

How can you expect someone to shower you with words of kindness and romantic adorations, if your own inner dialogue is scolding, critical and utterly unsupportive? Again, an impossible task. How can you dream of that evolved partner that understands and embodies the highest spiritual values, when you are distanced from your soul's essence, and out of touch with your purpose? No, precisely nothing will happen or worse yet, an entirely different person will show up, one that mirrors your weakness and magnifies your insecurities. For if he was the opposite and showered your with never-ending praise, how could you sustain that if you depended on his every word just to function?

You see, your love relationship begins actually long before your partner physically appears in your life. You set up the dynamics, you project your needs, your longings and well as your gifts to the world and if you are lacking self love, your partner will be a temporary one, teaching you the needed lessons and most often in painful ways. But if you lovingly work on every aspect of yourself, you will project such physical beauty, purity of your mind and light of your spirit that you will outshine all human limitations. And when your mind is clear, and filled with kind thoughts, gentle words and encouragement, your partner will be alike. And when your spirit is aligned with the universal truth and you are clear with your purpose and pure in intention, you will attract your absolute ultimate partner that will not only mirror your positive characteristics, but will magnify them, so together you become the dream pairing.

How can you get to that point? Awareness of your beautiful essence, its blessings and responsibilities, and the appreciative loving care you offer to yourself, will reward you with majestic power that will carry you thru anything. Allowing your body to relax and regenerate, nurturing it like you would a sweet baby, and listening to its needs, are the rules to obey and never ignore.

Train your mind to say what you decide, and not repeat those old critical patterns you may have heard in the past. And truly dedicate some time for inner reflection to understand who you are, your purpose, your needs, and know what makes you happy. It's unrealistic, unreasonable, and unfair to expect of your partner to make you happy. They won't, because they cannot; only you can. How do you expect to have fun with them if you can't have fun with yourself? Ask yourself; would you want to spend an entire day with you? Have a discussion or simply sit in silence, alone? Prepare a beautiful meal and laugh at something you read or observe, again alone? Learn to do that, become a fun person to be with, happy, peaceful and content.

If you want to hear that you are beautiful, first learn to say that to yourself and then see what happens. Now the partner that you long for in your life will only add to this idealistic picture. This way you won't be torn apart if they need some time alone, you won't be insecure if they don't grab your body every second of the day, and you won't cry childish fearful tears when everything does not revolve around you all the time. You won't need a partner out of desperation; you will want them out of love. Your ability for self-love decides whom you call into your life. So when this special person does appear out of the blue sky, they will be even indescribably more magical than you ever thought possible. And you won't have to do a thing but simply smile… and you'll both be in heaven.

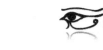

Friendship Love

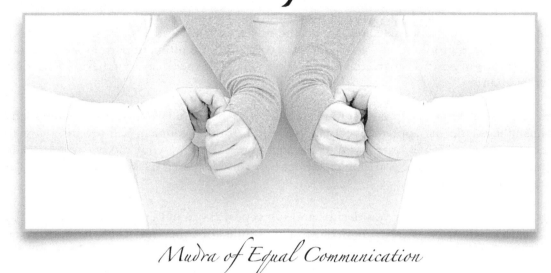

Mudra of Equal Communication

Love Mudras will help you deepen and expand your expression
of limitless Friendship, which will sustain your Love at all times.

Your partner should be your very closest, dearest, devoted, and most loving friend. One that you can trust with your life, and he will always save you. One that knows all your secrets, and he will never reveal or use them against you. One that knows your weaknesses and fears, and will never take advantage of them. One that knows your fantasies and dreams, and will help you achieve them. One that knows and understands your essence, and will never take advantage of it. One that knows your vulnerability, and will always protect you, the best he can. One that is reliable, and will always come through for you. One that knows and loves your heart, and will always unconditionally love you in return.

Is this possible? Actually, that depends on you. It depends on how you build your friendship. It depends on how honest you are with him, and if you allow him to visit the secret and sacred compartments of your heart and show him your Soul's brilliant light. And of course it depends on what kind of friend you are to him.

Are you capable of being his true unconditional friend? And if he told you the truth that you don't want to hear, would you still be his friend then? A true friend does not judge - and when he makes a decision you don't like or approve of, can you go beyond it and remain his loyal ally?

A true friend does not punish - and if he made a mistake and you got hurt, would you play games to seek revenge or would you remain steady in forgiveness if he asked you for it? A true friend does not push you into decisions you may not want - and if he made a choice that does not include your wishes, could you overcome the bitter disappointment and remain stoic and strong in your friendship? A true friend showers you with love even when the world turns against you - are you capable of remaining the last one standing when the world deserts him and he has no power, name, strength and no friends? A true friend will recognize when you are broken and weak, and will come and pick you up from the ashes and nurture you back to life, even if it was unpleasant, boring and most inconvenient.

Are you able to sacrifice your comfort and offer him that? A true friend does not care what others say about you or if it is not beneficial to have your association - would you be able to ignore the pressure, stand guard and protect him from enemy's attacks? A true friend will remain with you through the years even when you are less successful, beautiful, vibrant, wealthy, famous or desirable - are you able to overcome these accolades and stay by his side for the humble stripped-down version of him? A true friend respects your wishes to live or die - and even if your agony of loosing him overwhelms you, are you able to grant him his last wish? A true friend will never desert you, leave you alone to suffer in silence, and let you down when you most need him. Would you cross the seven seas to come pull him out of despair and give him hope? A true friend accepts you even if you cannot give him what he wants; he accepts your imperfections, oddities, annoying tiresome habits, your time wasting nonsense, overdramatic outbursts and useless complaints. Can you tolerate that and be patient while he goes thru this journey? A true friend will be there for you thru thick and thin, thru glory and loss, thru joy and pain, sorrow and sadness, laughter and tears - will you do that for him?

A true friend takes time to understand, feel and respect your essence - are you willing to sacrifice your precious time, patience, and seek within your Soul to grasp his spiritual depth? And if he told you the harshest of truths, that he does not love you any more like a lover does, and you'd break into a thousand irreparable pieces - would you still be able to remain his friend? If the answer is yes, then you understand what true unconditional Friendship Love is.

But if a person can not offer you kindness, compassion, loyalty and trust, you should distance yourself from them and know that your true friend is yet to come. And when he does, he will stand by your side, protect your heart and cherish every singular second with you - for there is only one of you. Your true friend that loves and cares for you will never desert you, for he is a gift, a blessing and a direct messenger of the gods.

Love at First Sight

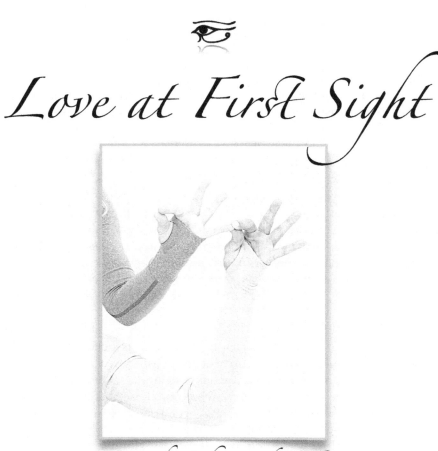

Mudra of Higher Understanding

Love Mudras will help you recognize and understand
your true destined Mate when connecting for the first time.

I believe that everyone who has the gift of experiencing love at first sight, understands that this can be a defining moment in your life. An instantaneous energy shift occurs and there is no denying that consequences will follow. If you recognize this moment, I suggest you acknowledge it with all your heart.

Love at first sight has many different flavors. The less desirable is when it stings you instantaneously and infuses you with a feeling of hypnotic imbalance as well as foreboding sense that you are descending down a path that could be quite dangerous, and your heart could get wounded, perhaps mortally. But you still follow your heart's call and throw yourself into the unknown, despite your Soul's suspicion and haunting knowing that this particular experience will be a painful and learning one, and not the one where you happily ride off together into the sunset. There will be challenges, tests and eventual separation, for this was the purpose of it all.

Then there is the other, good "love at first sight" kind, where you actually do not feel any fear or pain, but an instantaneous unmistakable energetic recognition of your partner when you first see, hear or interact with them. A very powerful yet peaceful magnetic pull persistently stays with you and affects you in a most profound way. Hopefully your Soul recognizes and understands this "first sight" attraction, but its fulfillment depends on how fearful or cooperative you are.

If your heart is still recovering from a painful experience, if your mind is trying to find logical arguments against it, if your physical body is all detached in frozen fear of your past, you may try to find a million reasons and explanations why this may not be true love since there is no pain, and no deep longing infused with a grain of sadness and hurt.

Does love have to hurt to be real?
No, for it is only in karmic unresolved love where the experience is intertwined with the pain of learning and growing process for you, whereas in a harmonious "love at first sight" you will feel a sense of deep heart connection, profound mutual trust, respect and understanding, familiar safety and perhaps even far away clarity, that this is the person meant for you, as unusual or impossible as that may seem. Depending on your previous experiences and what your heart has endured, you may need some time to truly open up and allow this healthy love to manifest and live. However, the fact that you attracted it into your life shows that you are more ready than you dare to admit.

Some of us have a tendency to romanticize this experience, perhaps throwing ourselves into the wild ocean of love, not even thinking about the possibility of waves drowning us. And when after a broken heart you find yourself wounded and washed ashore, you believe that "love at first sight" will never happen to you again, or you associate it with the pain of an unavoidable broken heart, and perhaps it's not possible, and everything is just a fairy tale. But in fact if you remain energetically open, your true destined partner will appear and you will know it in that precise instant.

It will be "Love at first sight" yet it may not frighten you, or steal your peace, but a different, much lovelier, warm, familiar and incredibly comforting feeling will envelop you, for deep down in your soul you will know that this indeed is your destined equal partner and yes, they are here at last. The energy pull will be so profound you won't be able to resist, and their overwhelming love will open you up like a flower to a seeking butterfly and then…your life will truly never be the same. Does that sound too romantic? Perhaps, but I insist that it is possible.

Karmic Love

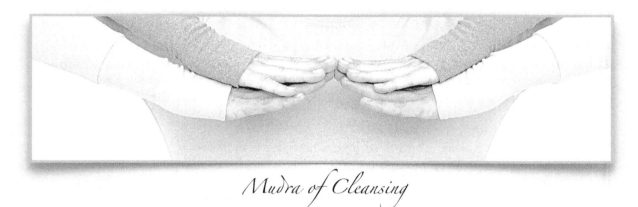

Mudra of Cleansing

*Love Mudras will help you cleanse and release old experiences,
so you may open your Heart and create space for your True Love.*

The wheel of Karma is a complex, intricate and non-negotiable one. And since love is the ultimate energy of the Universe, the lessons of the heart affect us to the core.

Karmic love has different manifestations, and yes, most likely it is an unresolved connection that teaches you thru a painful experience. But karmic love can also be a very harmonious bond from the past, with no dues or debts, but with an already earned credit to help you both expedite your human experience in this lifetime so you can arrive at the true home of your essence.

However, karmic love burdened with debts is like a training ground, a previously agreed upon experience to learn in an expedited manner.

Hopefully such experience will help you prepare for your true destined ultimate partner, so that you can eventually soar to the sky, limitless and free.

The one characteristic with debt ridden karmic love is that you truly cannot avoid it; it will show up like an uninvited stranger disrupting your seemingly peaceful uneventful life, creating an instant change, confusion and upheaval. It will break-up previous seemingly harmonious but stagnant relationships, it will propel you to do crazy dangerous things, to risk it all and have a complete disregard for the fragility of your heart. You will break your unwritten rules, shock yourself with your expanded tolerance, your never-ending ability for forgiveness and your willingness to stand on the edge, ready to throw yourself off the cliff at a moments notice, just to make your lover happy.

If you are a born pleaser this will be your weakest link. And when you realize for the millionth time that your lover doesn't feel like you, that their love has conditions, that you never were, are, or will be their priority, then you begin to crumble. Often the decision how long you will allow this charade to go on depends on your ability to stand up for yourself, learn to love yourself enough and embrace the fact that you do in fact deserve better.

Your initial shock that you don't seem to be enough for your lover in whatever context, this is the hardest lesson to learn. How is it possible that you gave the very best of you and it still was not enough? How could you fail so drastically and completely? Once you gather your strength, and save yourself with a jump off the roller coaster, your true deep inner work begins. And yes, you may need a few more rounds, you may wait while your heart aches and bruised ego hopes for this karmic lover to realize what they lost and come running after you in the middle of a stormy night, crying and begging for another chance. And yes, you may grant them that, only to see awfully fast that nothing has changed.

And when you make the final break and allow your heart the freedom and air to breathe and hopefully create some space for a new loving soul to come into your life, your karmic partner may realize just what they wasted and lost. They may lament for years how you were their biggest love, how sorry they are, how they wish they had you back. Can you listen to your heart and disregard your ego's vanity? Can you remain strong enough in your self-love to resist this old song that you longed to hear in the past?

Can you recognize their habit of wanting what they cannot have, how that always seems so much more desirable to them? And yes, you may always love them in a certain way, but with maturity, detached distance, and deeper clarity. You will gladly let them go, and will understand how all of it was indeed very necessary, how you gained knowledge, and are ready to stand in your core and attract a partner that will not make you suffer, beg and tolerate unacceptable behavior, but someone who will love you unconditionally, gently uplift you, kindly tend to your heart, and give you a sense of loyalty, complete trust and freedom to be who you truly are. Because you are amazing, just the way you are.

Physical-Sexual Love

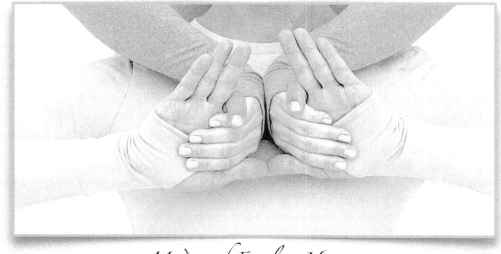

Mudra of Fearless Honesty

*Love Mudras will help you manifest and experience the expression
of Physical Love at the highest possible frequency level.*

Physical merging with your partner is a most powerful energy exchange that remains with you for a long while. You are opening yourself up to receive their essence in a most profound and direct way, you become affected by their frequency, their blending with your subtle core power and when your heart is fully open in this dynamic, you are most vulnerable. Your lover's strengths as well as needs linger within you, affect you, your energy field is wide open in trust, completely exposed and raw, unable to protect itself from any unharmonious exchange. You are giving your partner a full access to your essence, like a flower bloom offering it's mesmerizing scent.

Nowadays we are under steady pressure to look and act a certain way, and if you allow into your life a partner who sees only your physical body's assets, you will have to learn a difficult lesson, for you will be forced to chase time with persistent fury and yet you will never win or find peace.

If you are careless and not secure in your core, an energetically unbalanced physical exchange will deplete and affect you in a negative way. If your sense of self is tied solely to your physicality and your partner has no idea about your soul's essence, you are on a one-way ticket to nowhere. Therefore be very selective about whom you allow into you energy "orbit". Wasting your time with an inappropriate partner will prevent you from attracting, recognizing and opening up to your true love. Once you do meet your destined lover, take your time to establish a truly strong base, so that your sexual expression is the highest extension of mutual love, trust and honesty where all fear is diminished and your body and heart can open in a most loving way.

With this dynamic you will create a transformative magnified energy field that will sustain you much longer than your physical merging. But here is the catch: make sure that you are not the only one feeling this awakened core power and perhaps just wishing your partner was at the same energy frequency level as you. In fact, during the peak of the sexual act you may have experienced only your own ecstatic power and not that of the two merging equals. You may give yourself completely to your partner and they will certainly enjoy it, but after the actual sexual act you will be left empty and alone and not because they fell asleep, or dashed to their Iphone, but because they were never really there with you, certainly not on the level of consciousness you were.

They were simply lost in the furious desire for your flesh and you confused their physical passion for the ultimate act of unconditional love, where two equals physically merge and transform not only themselves, but also the world that surrounds them. Everyone that encounters such a pairing feels this exquisite unique bond of unbreakable love. You see, the physical attraction between two people will change, transform and perhaps even completely disappear if there is no other glue holding them together.

From an energetic perspective the kundalini power that sleeps at the base of your spine is a most powerful bond and if only one partner has an awakened kundalini power and the other one is still "asleep", it will be most disappointing for the advanced partner to realize that in fact they misunderstood the act of physical love for a higher, deeper connection.

Therefore, before you share the luxury of your sexual love energy, be highly selective and you will see, once you merge with your true equal, you will never doubt about it, you will never suffer or cry about it except tears of pure bliss, because in the land of true unconditional love, there is no separation or turning back, for your love is an eternal joint entity that was, is, and will remain with both of you forever more.

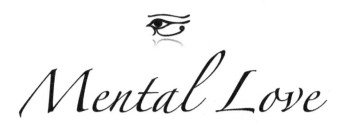

Mental Love

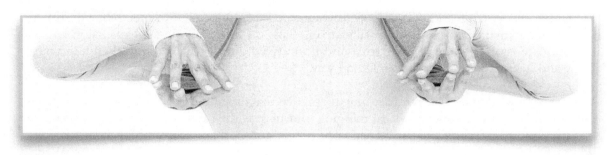

Mudra of Perfect Mental Balance

*Love Mudras will calm and focus your mind into a state of stillness,
which will activate your synchronicity and silent communication.*

No matter how powerful your physical, emotional and spiritual attraction is, do not underestimate the power of synchronicity, compatibility and love between your minds. Yes, your physical and energy bodies respond to an energetic pull, but your mind is not far behind in translating and associating it with familiar perceptions and criteria.

While I believe that spiritual love frequency within your energy body is the true doorway to your essence, your mind certainly has a lot to say. It is with your mind that you recall exciting memories of times past, dream up beautiful moments of your future, and it is your mind that constantly accompanies you at this very precise moment.

What is your mind's commentary right now? You see, it has something to say, almost all the time.

When two lovers connect deeply and completely, they experience a startling synchronicity of their minds. They can finish each other's sentences, think alike, and communicate without uttering a word.

This perfect collaboration and love attunement of your minds creates an even more powerful energy dynamic between the two of you and when this is manifested at the highest level of clarity, inner focus, and the purest of thoughts filled with deep compassion, respect and love for one another, you two become somewhat unbeatable and frighteningly magnetic. You stop others in their tracks and people feel an invisible pull towards the two of you, wanting to be near you to experience this tangible magic that surrounds you.

Mental love also means clarity about each other's wishes, fantasies, desires and support for each other in most selfless ways. The unconditional dynamic infused into this experience gives each one of you the freedom to be who you want, pursue what your heart desires, but more than that. With the support of your partner, their trust and belief in your abilities you become invincible, fueled by energy of such magnitude that no obstacle is too big to conquer, and no limitation too impossible to overcome.

It is essential that your partner is self-confident and recognizes that you truly are a team and that no matter what, they will stand by you, offer a consoling word, a loving hug and a rescuing hand if you ever get lost at sea. They will be there with advice, encouraging words to infuse you with hope when you feel weak and broken. That is true partnership, when your partner will celebrate your accomplishments and help you reach further, they will watch your back and never fear that if you are strong and resilient they may lose you, if the world sees your beauty someone may steal you, or you will escape them, or when you succeed you may replace them.

For you never will - you see, such a partner is truly irreplaceable and your achievements will be magnified with them by your side and not hampered by their insecure fears and competitive desperation. And if their behavior is to the contrary, this will be the first emergency alarm warning you that they may not be your true love destined partner. Your partner should be mindful when discovering the treasures of your physical temple, expressing their emotions, and open minded in joint stillness when you reach for spiritual otherworldly secrets.
In your minds you can share your wildest fantasies and dreams and travel anywhere, anytime, regardless of limitations known to our physical existence. Together in your mind, you can envision and ultimately create your future, and consciously open the last gate to your heart, trusting your true love. Your minds are your sacred swords that overcome all obstacles and help you consciously expand your awareness and receptivity to otherworldly information.

Having mental synchronicity can be almost as exciting as making physical love, perhaps not quite, but almost. And imagine having both! Your mind is your "love organ", much more powerful than you can imagine. Merging minds create pure ecstatic bliss.

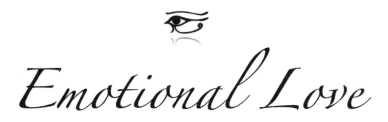

Emotional Love

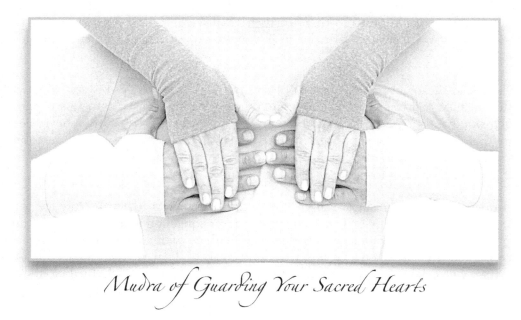

Mudra of Guarding Your Sacred Hearts

*Love Mudras will help you fine tune your hearts to function
in perfect harmony, trust and magnified power or equal exchange.*

The power of emotions is not to be used lightly. Like the irresistible current of a wild ocean, the emotions will pull you into directions unknown, unwanted, and out of control. Emotions are most difficult to tame and will twirl you around, spin you relentlessly and possibly hurl you far into the distance without a safe place to land. When you can't manage your emotions, you are very vulnerable, weak and unstable. And when you can't harness your overall emotional state in a love relationship, then anything is possible.

You see, once that sacred love-key unlocks the door to your heart, everything flows out in spades and you better be ready. Here comes the reality check of how prepared, mature and in touch with yourself you truly are. If you have not done any work on yourself and have just piled all your emotions into that secret compartment in the far away corner of your heart, this one day when you fall in love, you will experience quite a tornado.

The transformative power of love is non-negotiable and of such nature, that your heart will be unable to withstand it and pretend all is sorted out and in perfect harmony. In fact the entire cascade of old, unresolved emotions will eventually explode and escape your carefully guarded fortress. In a weak moment of self-doubt, the wall will break down.

Old hurt, insecurities, fears, anger, neediness, guilt, just to name a few favorite ones, all will line up and want their day in the sun - within your relationship. So while your partner views in shock some completely other person that suddenly appeared, you will be battling and hushing up all these uninvited guests, or more likely permanent residents of your heart, that you never acknowledged, but denied and ignored. Now they want your attention and they will get it. But the price will be high, for your partner will not like and certainly not love all these other versions of you that make you look like a stranger and nothing like the person they knew and adored. Therefore it is essential that you know yourself, acknowledge and reconcile with all your emotions before you open up and make space for a loved one to enter into your life. Once you accomplish this task, you are perfectly ready to reveal your heart to someone else, pure and open, without restrictions, unresolved fears and burdens.

Emotional love of such a pure nature is an incredible elixir of endless energy and inspiration, magnifying your natural gifts, expanding your loving abilities and delivering you at the threshold of most precious adventure, meaning unconditional love. You see, until your own emotions are understood, you won't be able to experience this life changing development. If the emotions of love trigger fear, your every decision, choice, expression, and word will be tied with this precise emotion and your lover won't hear your true heart. They will hear your fear, which is not the real, beautiful and pure essence of you.

Once you are free of all those extensive tentacles of old sorrow and hurt, you are ripe for the ultimate expression of the most substantial emotion of them all - love without boundaries or limitations. Love is the greatest and superior emotion of them all, for without love there is nothing. Once you understand love in all its glory, you will accept and recognize how significant this consciousness is in every aspect of your life and your soul's evolution.

Embrace your emotions with a delicate touch, talk to them sweetly, and thank them for coming into your life. They teach you who you are and reveal the natural shades of being a human being. And then, let them go so you can become whole and free. Your true love partner awaits, open the gates and let them in, so they may listen to the ethereal sound of your pure heart.

True Unconditional Love

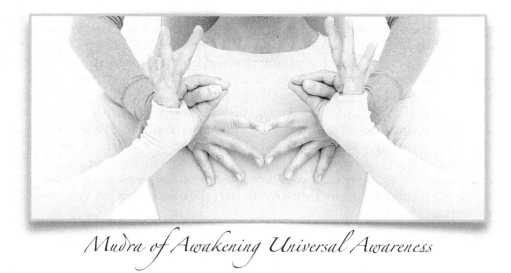

Mudra of Awakening Universal Awareness

*Love Mudras will help you develop and live in everlasting
and unbreakable Unconditional Love of the highest manifestation.*

When you are a natural giver, you want to give freely, openly and without limitations. If this is in your true essence, you will always remain this way. I do not believe that this characteristic is prevalent in a woman or a man, I believe that it depends purely on the soul and its evolutionary state. Even if on your life's journey you meet people that are unkind, take advantage of you, and wound you while hurling a toxic arrow of selfishness right into the center of your giving heart, you will remain who you are - a giver from the heart.

Yes, in the aftermath of a disappointment you shall suffer, cry and hide in the cave while you lick your wounds and wonder why this world is so full of darkness, and how is it possible that someone you gave everything to, just did not understand the pure concept of it. But if your nature is truly giving, you will also be for-giving and will understand that such a person was simply not capable of comprehending such love, and could not help himself but take advantage of your extended hand offering them pure golden nuggets.

They loved you to the best of their capacities, but that was so far removed from your own ability to love, that the incompatibility was of galactic irreconcilable proportions. You may still love them, but from a distance and in an entirely different way, like you would love a being of a different species, with awareness that they are simply incapable of love interaction on your level.

It is human nature to be suspicious or wary, always wondering where the enemy is hiding and what is expected of us. Therefore we often misunderstand the concept of unconditional love as contrary to the need of self preservation and survival, cultivating the feeling of required conditions in love, otherwise we fear someone would take complete advantage of us while we gave them no conditions or rules to obey.

Another expected dynamic is the expectation of a return for our investment of "giving" love. In fact, in love there should be no expectations or need for rules and restrictions, because if you truly love someone in an unconditional way, you will not consider such an absurd action as to taking advantage of them, dishonesty, irresponsibility or unkindness. These concepts do not exist in the realm of unconditional love. They exist in the world of limited love, filled with fears, insecurities, anger, old pain, and helpless participation in situations that multiply and repeat all these negative manifestations.Unconditional love is only possible when the individual has acquired the ability to give generously, truly without any expectations whatsoever, and has overcome any selfish tendencies, and all related habits that keep our souls entrapped on this earthly realm.

When you are an unselfish, generous and kindhearted partner and lover, you are ready to move on, for you truly don't belong to this world anymore, since it is not aligned with your core frequency. Once you meet your destined partner that resonates with you in every possible way, you are granted the exclusive opportunity to ascend and enter the world where unconditional love is the currency that rules. Now you are ascending into supernatural existence.

When two lovers that are both equally capable of unconditional love meet, an immense shift occurs. They become examples of giving each other every nuance of human love manifestation, intertwined with tenderness, kindness, attentiveness, exquisite attunement to each other and absolute loyal devotion. The trust and passion of this coupling is the optimal experience of a human love relationship. These two souls have a profoundly deep connection, reaching into the far past and extending into the distant future, for they belong to the very exquisitely fortunate people that found their soul-mate or twin flame.

Soul Mates & Twin Flames

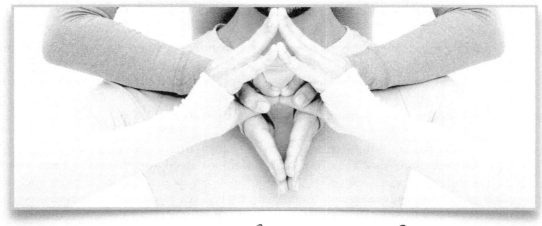

Mudra of Heaven on Earth

*Love Mudras will help you attract, recognize and accomplish
your Soul's primary mission of returning Home with your equal other half.*

It seems that nowadays the world is filled with people searching for their soulmates. It is like an epidemic, a desperate effort that seems so futile and impossible to accomplish. In this search, the seeker is equipped with sky high expectations, for they imagine that this soulmate will have all the answers to their questions and will resolve every singular problem they have had, or will encounter in their future.

The expectation of this soulmate before they ever step thru the door is overwhelming. Of course, the seeker usually spends much less time seeking for their own answers or getting to know themselves in the first place. They are sadly unaware that it is precisely their inner confusion and frazzled message to the universe which is preventing this desired meeting from occurring. Simple answer; you are not ready. Long answer; find out who you are, what you want, what you have to offer, learn to be happy, fulfilled and self sufficient in your emotional state and then…maybe you will be a step closer to a healthy and balanced equally proportioned relationship. There is just no way around it, the fact is there is no shortcut to true soulmate love.

A soul mate is someone very special for they are amazingly compatible with you, they truly understand you, feel the same way about various life views and possibly have the same interests. We can have numerous soulmates that we meet thru our life, and they do not have to be our lovers. A really close dear friend can be your soulmate and you love each other dearly in the natural dynamic of friendship - love.

A union with a soulmate is usually a content and happy one, you may accomplish desired life missions and feel true love and support for one another. However this is not the highest manifestation of love. Why not? Because the one sacred element is missing, and that is complete and indisputable synchronicity of body, mind, heart and spirit. It is like the difference between vacationing in a wonderful first class hotel or relishing your true home. In the case of a soulmate, everything is there, all the luxuries and comforts, entertainment, fantastic food and truly anything you wish for. But you know the whole time one indisputable fact; that you are not in the irreplaceable comfort and safety of your home. You are visiting, temporarily, and you can pretend that right now you do live there, but you know this is not your true heart's domain.

If you are so fortunate and divinely blessed, that one predestined day, you encounter a being perfectly and extraordinarily alike yourself, your life will never be the same. It is like the previously crooked and seemingly unchangeable galaxy suddenly realigned itself into pure perfection of an order. It is like someone is so much like you that it simply takes your breath away. And when this happens, you may get frightened or stand in disbelief trying to find reasons and explanations why this could not possibly work or even be true. Surely any moment you will see that this person is not as perfect as they seem. And you wait, and wait. And then you realize that they are really here, standing beside you and giving you that sense that you longed for with every cell of you body. The absolute irrevocable consistent feeling that your heart is finally home. And in fact it does not matter where you reside or travel or move to. The feeling persist wherever you are and never ceases to leave you.

You have met your Twin flame and together you are in perfect synchronicity and symphony.Of course, your reaction to your first encounter may be different. You will recognize them in an instant like a lightning bolt out of nowhere. You will know this is it, in a million inexplicable words and matching floating emotions that will descend upon your body with a gentle caress. And suddenly a new sensation will emerge, straight from the center of your heart. It will unravel and light you up in a way you never knew it could, and with such power and might you'll be transformed forever. This extraordinary experience will ignite an instant recognition and frequency synthesis that will merge you two into a new, even more compelling entity. Your hearts will be de-cyphered and upgraded into an entirely new constellation. There is no return from this occurrence, for this process is irreversible, otherworldly, and of too subtle nature for this coarse, earthly realm.

However, the consequences will be felt and revealed in both of your lives almost instantaneously. Your merged power will have an indescribably transformative effect on anyone and everything that approaches the orbit of your unified alliance. Your combined frequencies will have an everlasting influence on environment and anything you touch will be permeated with your unique joint substance of this majestic and otherworldly Love flame.

Why is this combination so forceful and otherworldly? Because the ultimate energy of the universe is unconditional love of such massive proportions that we can not comprehend its concept or magnitude. When a spark of that force is reconnected in two beings alike, the strength is amplified, unimaginably so. When this moment occurs and you've met your Twin flame, an invisible clock will be set in motion and your time on this earth will be your last.

However, there is a secret code that needs to be in place in order for all of this to occur. You see, the greatest mystery of the Twin flame manifestation in your life is the fact that before you can reconnect with your Twin flame, you need to reconnect the Twin flames within you. It is your complete inner balance, your self love and unconditional acceptance of yourself that will help you accomplish that. Releasing old fears, old attachments, and truly listening to your heart and soul. Yes, the answer to the puzzle of unconditional Twin flame love is right in your essence. Does that mean that you don't need to or will never meet your Twin flame?

I simply means that your inner ethereal energy makings are so complex and yet self-supportive that you need to understand this perfectly complete configuration of the Twin flame energy within you, before you are truly ready for your Twin flame partner. So while you may or may not connect with your Twin flame partner in this lifetime, you can ascend into the higher realms of existence and it could be precisely there that your Twin flame partner awaits. Thus each one of us needs to be whole, to ignite the Twin flame within and when you do blend with your Twin flame partner in unconditional love, your power is unimaginable. This meeting is predestined, previously agreed upon and may happen on any realm of existence. The vibratory rate of your re-union is mighty powerful and transformative when used for helping and raising consciousness of others.

This ultimate reward distinctly implies you have completed your journey's assignments and are ready to truly and deeply understand the next dimension, the other side, the side we can not see, hear or touch from here, for it is finer than a summer breeze and brighter than the fresh new snow. It is in fact brilliance in motion, transcending in your ecstatic unconditional love and bliss.

Mudras for Two

~ Practice sets ~

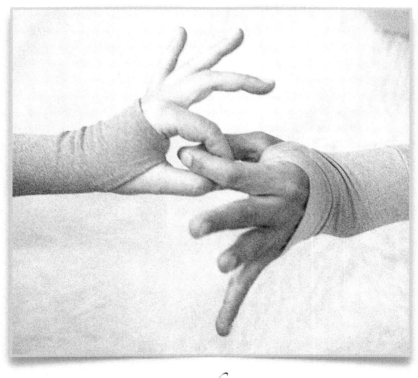

Mudra of Creation

Part Three

Align Your Body

My temple is my greatest treasure while here on earth.
It offers me a safe haven for my soul to reside in, and precious gifts
so I can marvel at the beauty of nature and all earthly creation.
And it gives me a rare opportunity to experience your love thru the eyes of a lover, friend, companion and ally.
When we master all these incarnations and learn to love with our hearts,
we are brought back together, to unite once more on our journey home.
Yes, it is beautiful here, but incomparable to the beauty of Us.

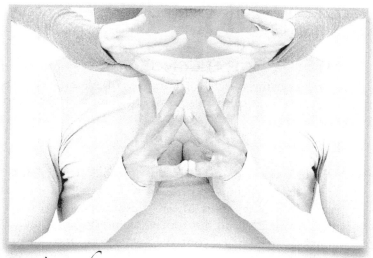

Mudra of Opening & Merging Two Hearts

MUDRA *for* CHAKRA I.

DYNAMICS

The communication and assurance each partner needs, is not based on purely materialistic issues. The core energies permeate much deeper nuances of relationship dynamics than the expected physical manifestations. Despite the obvious, individuals with material riches can spend their entire lives feeling insecure about their survival or sense of support and protection from their partner. On the other side of the spectrum, a couple that lives in modest circumstances can enjoy absolute harmony and domestic bliss, because they truly mastered this energy dynamic and created a strong and solid base regardless of their financial affluence. These subtle energy needs, are much more substantial than what meets the eye. A woman can feel wonderfully protected simply by the loving nearness of her partner, regardless of his material wealth. Likewise, the man can feel nurtured and strongly supported by his partner who creates a warm and loving home base - their foundation.

WEAKNESS AND IMBALANCE

Disharmony and incompatibility in this chakra center can create conflict with the following dynamics: instability or unequal disposition towards material wealth, lack of generosity and sharing of material possessions, restrictive behavior of the materially stronger partner, difficulty in feeling grounded and unified as a couple, incompatible disposition towards the financial future, general lack of vitality and energy force in relationship, disconnection from nature and healthy lifestyle habits. These disfavored dynamics will result in negative consequences strongly affecting the next, as well as all other chakras.

CHALLENGE

If you find yourself in a relationship purely for purposes of material security and safety, be aware that you will not advance in a spiritual sense until you overcome fears that keep you in such a dysfunctional dynamic.

REMEDY

You can improve and magnify vital energy levels in this chakra by clearly communicating and immediately noticing and voicing individual wishes and concerns. If you feel disappointed in your partner's disposition in any of these aspects, it is most important that you speak about it openly and clearly, and not remain silent, hoping they will come to their senses. The longer you wait, the deeper your dissatisfaction, and the harder will be to achieve positive changes. The sooner you speak the better chances you have of establishing a healthy, balanced dynamic that you desire. Create a stable home environment, develop healthy habits, make time for activities that promote connectedness, nurture a respectful disposition regardless of earthly possessions, cultivate nonjudgmental views, talk about mutual goals that encompass wishes of both. This will help establishing a sense of togetherness and mutual trust and support. Simple changes, like saying "we" instead of "I" give the partner immediate sense of equal ground and common interests for a positive, united and stronger future. This shift will magnify your power of manifestation with great force and velocity.

ASPECTS ~ Vitality, survival, security, willpower, foundation, courage
LOCATION ~Base of spine
COLOR ~ Red
SENSE ~ Smell

Speak from Your Heart:

"I will protect you. You are safe with me. I give you my strength and security."

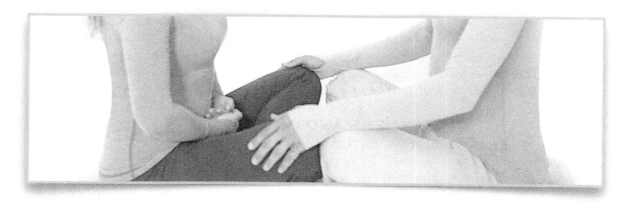

Sit with a straight back and face your partner, knees touching lightly. Place your hands in your lap, left hand resting in right, with palms relaxed and facing up towards the sky. Your partner will place his hands on your knees, offering energy support, a sense of stability and protection. The energy flow from his hands will travel directly towards your first chakra center and help create a supportive energy base.

Breath is long, deep and slow. Gaze in your partner's eyes, projecting love, openness and trust. Practice for three minutes. Now <u>reverse</u> the positions, your partner resting his hands in his lap, left hand in right, palms turned up towards the sky. Now place your hands on his knees, and offer nurturing, supportive and loving energy. Gently with loving kindness look deeply into each other's eyes, project love and trusting support in complete unity, equality and respect. Practice for three minutes.

Affirmation:

I AM YOUR PILLAR OF STRENGTH, SUPPORT AND SAFETY.

MUDRA for CHAKRA 2.

DYNAMICS

The communication and assurance each partner needs in this case, is not based purely on needs of a sexual nature. The core energy of second chakra plays an essential part in creative expression of all kinds. Supporting this facet of a personality is essential for inner fulfillment and satisfaction, as well as one's acceptance of all forms of creativity. Creative expression is a highly therapeutic modality and heals numerous afflictions. By acknowledging one's creative desires you harmonize and positively affect also the nature of sexual expression, which can as a consequence exalt and evolve into the highest form of physical communication on that level. Our sexual identity is a very fragile aspect as is our creative nature. A very important choice is the role of a compatible partner, who can help us mature and learn to fully express our creative nature. Sexual passion is short lived if there is no substance and substantial energetic bond. Once such bond is nurtured and treasured, the physical aspect of love serves its purpose of offering the opportunity for two individuals to experience true synergy of souls and transcend the limited sensory abilities of this world.

WEAKNESS AND IMBALANCE

Disharmony and incompatibility in this chakra center can create conflict with the following dynamics: exploiting the partner as a physical object of desire without emotional participation, manipulation of others, jealousy, restlessness, addiction and anxiety, all resulting in dishonesty and escapism. These disfavored dynamics will result in negative consequences strongly affecting the next - third, as well as all other chakras.

CHALLENGE

If you find yourself in a relationship based on purely physical needs of a sexual nature, be aware that you will not advance in a spiritual sense until you overcome these emotionally disconnected and addictive tendencies that keep you in such a dysfunctional dynamic.

REMEDY

Communicating your needs and desires clearly. Awareness of your partner' s sensitivities, wishes, as well as passions. Respecting personal dispositions and preferences that may differ from yours. Expressing appreciation for one another, developing deep trust, and surrendering to one another without fear or inhibitions. Kindness and understanding of partner's wounds and fragility. Openness to exploring unique expressions of creativity. Establishing a new healthy interplay, healing the past and expressing loving, compassionate and affectionate gentleness towards one another. Supporting your partner's pursuit of creative expression. Preventing stagnation, exploring new and dedicating regular and committed time to one another.

ASPECTS ~ Creativity, sex, procreation, family, inspiration
LOCATION ~Sex Organs
COLOR ~ Orange
SENSE ~ Taste

Speak from Your Heart:

"You are beautiful, you are everything I desire and want, I admire your creativity."

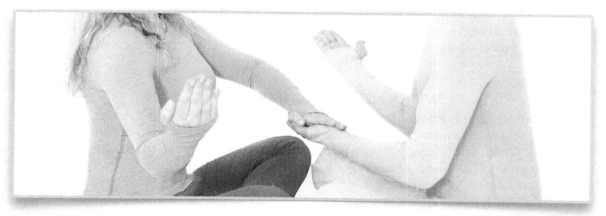

Sit with a straight back and face your partner, knees almost touching. Lift the right hand to shoulder level away from the body and to the side. Palm is facing up towards the sky. Lift the left hand and place it palm down on your partner's open left palm that is facing up. In this Mudra, the woman's hand is on top, as the manifestation of the feminine, ascending energy.

Breath is long, deep and slow. Look into your partner's eyes and see the divine creative power in him. Project unconditional love and admiration for every moment you two are fortunate to be sharing together. Practice for three minutes.

Affirmation:

WE ENTER OUR TEMPLE OF LOVE WITH RESPECT
AND UNCONDITIONAL LOVE.

MUDRA *for* CHAKRA 3.

DYNAMICS

The communication and assurance each partner needs in this case, hold multiple and complex aspects that affect every area of your relationship. This is in fact the most challenging chakra center to evolve from and finally ascend into the heart center. Anger and fear rule this center and any kind of serious imbalance with these emotions will be very unfavorable in your relationship. The energies that hold you hostage here are tightly intertwined with ego and mind, and unless you learn to control these aspects, they will control you and take over your life, and your relationship dynamics. When you remain in conflict with your partner out of principle, stubbornness, pride, vanity, your ego is in charge. Overcoming an overly dominant ego and issues of control are supremely important when it comes to relationships, and both partners can help each other recognize as well as transform these negative habits and tendencies. On the positive side, this center reflects the power of your will, the mind, and determination to accomplish a desired task or mission.

WEAKNESS AND IMBALANCE

Disharmony and incompatibility in this chakra center can create conflict with the following dynamics: control through authority or threat of anger, manipulation of power, misuse of fears, intimidation when not giving in, evoking feelings of guilt, selfishness, need for power, obsession with recognition. These disfavored dynamics will result in negative consequences strongly affecting the next - fourth, as well as all other chakras. When stuck in this center you will not be able to break out of "earthly entrapment" or evolve into the heart center of higher frequency.

CHALLENGE

If you find yourself in a relationship based on fear, ego power, or selfishness, be aware that you will not advance in a spiritual sense until you overcome these manipulative and ego caused negative tendencies that keep you in such a dysfunctional dynamic.

REMEDY

Honest, peaceful, direct, fearless and open communication when fear or ego threatens to take over the relationship. Kindness and encouragement for your partner, protecting each other from harm or negative influences, people, or surroundings. Never taking advantage of your partner's shortcomings, fears or weaknesses. Addressing anger and immediately working to resolve all conflicts of the day, not allowing negative situations to linger on. Offering each other complete support, helping each other overcome fears and eliminating issues of control. Instead of using power for your own selfish needs, learning to offer selfless support and empower your partner in a most generous and kindhearted way possible.

ASPECTS ~ Ego, emotional center, the intellect, the mind
LOCATION ~Solar Plexus
COLOR ~ Yellow
SENSE ~ Sight

Speak from Your Heart:

"Let go of fear, you are safe. I am with you and will protect you. No one will harm you."

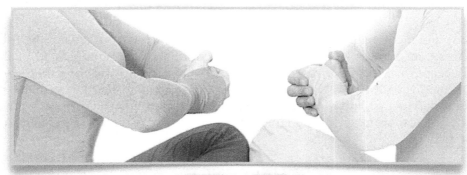

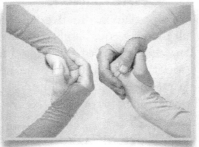

Sit with a straight back facing your partner, your knees touching lightly. Lift the hands up to the level of your heart, create a fist with the left hand and wrap your right hand around it. This Mudra for relaxation and joy will help you let go of any negative feelings that need to be released and are blocking a healthy flow of positive energy between you. Breathe land hold for three minutes and look deeply and lovingly into your partner's eyes.
Breathe long, deep and slow. Gaze into your partner's eyes with trust, unconditional love and kindness. Project complete acceptance and devotion. Practice for three minutes.

Affirmation:

WE ARE FEARLESS, LOYAL AND
EQUALS IN BODY, MIND AND SPIRIT.

MUDRA *for* CHAKRA 4.

DYNAMICS

The communication and assurance each partner needs in this case, is of a different nature. This chakra center is the first energy space that is considerably more removed from earthly existence and its limitations. Main challenge happens when one partner is incapable of and therefore incompatible in regards to unconditional love. Be aware that you will not be able to forcibly push your less spiritually evolved partner to ascend and make progress. Instead, the interaction will force you to descend and function at their lower level frequency. The only way to ascension is at ones own time and pace, most likely in another lifetime. Therefore this chakra is known as the "gate into higher consciousness".

WEAKNESS AND IMBALANCE

Disharmony and incompatibility in this chakra center can create conflict and the following consequences: unrequited love, unreturned affection, lack of compassion, failure to receive or accept love from partner, weakness of overextending and forgetting your own needs, extremely giving nature and generosity to inappropriate partner, inability to love yourself, self-destructive behavior, betrayal, taking for granted your partner's ability for forgiveness, imbalance in giving and receiving love between partners, inability to love unconditionally.

CHALLENGE

If you find yourself in a relationship lacking in deeper understanding of compassion, without kindness, and most of all missing equal ability to love unconditionally, you will be forced to let go, accept and learn your lesson of allowing and attracting a partner who is deserving of your love. Only proper compatibility on the heart level will offer you both the fulfillment you are seeking, complete and deep happiness of heart, and opportunity to ascend further in your spiritual evolutionary process.

REMEDY

Be acutely aware of your own needs and abilities. If your partner is not capable of understanding and offering true unconditional love, and yet you decide to remain with them, you need to respect your own soul's evolutionary placement and tend to your process of ascension. In such a case you can not expect to experience unconditional love. But if you have attracted into your life a compatible partner, you can further develop your abilities, by generously expressing love for one another. Practice conscious giving and receiving, openness and complete trust, dedication and support for each other, understanding and embracing each other's wishes without judgment or expectations. Stay unequivocally compassionate and reliable in your acts of kindness, and remain patient and supportive in all aspects of your partner's personal development and needs. Practice unconditional love each and every day in every possible way. If both partners are synchronized at this level, they will not experience serious conflicts.

ASPECTS ~ Unconditional true love, devotion, faith, compassion, self-love
LOCATION ~Heart
COLOR ~ Green & Pink
SENSE ~ Touch

Speak from Your Heart:

" I open my heart so that Our hearts may become One. I love you deeply and forever."

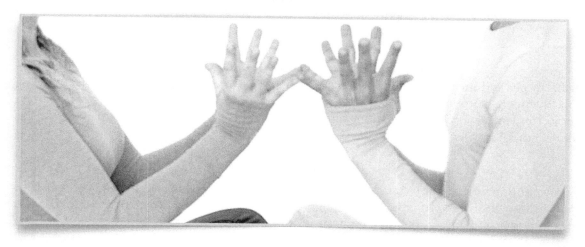

Sit with a straight back and face your partner, knees touching lightly. Lift up your hands and hold them in front of your heart, all fingers stretched and spread apart like a flower, your wrists are touching and only fingertips of little fingers are touching with your partner's little fingertips. Breathe and gaze into each other's eyes. Look into the heart and soul of your partner. See his divinity. Practice for three minutes and project unconditional love.

Breath is long, deep and slow.

Gaze into your partner's eyes, project unconditional love and an open heart.

Affirmation:

**OUR UNCONDITIONAL LOVE ENVELOPS US
BELOW, ABOVE AND WITHIN.**

MUDRA for CHAKRA 5.

DYNAMICS

Communication is the key player for this energy center and if you are energetically compatible you will experience much more than truthful, open and loving exchange between the two of you. In fact, this energy combustion and synchronization will offer you the unique opportunity to - as a couple - communicate to others and deeply affect them with your words of inspiration, motivation and enlightenment. This relationship will be based on deep, bonded and highly articulate communication. Such two souls alike, functioning with similar interest and aspirations, will become highly in tune with deeper spiritual knowledge and wisdom that will penetrate to the heart of the listener, while transforming the space and energy of their surroundings in a most positive and enlightening way.

WEAKNESS AND IMBALANCE

Disharmony and incompatibility in this chakra center can create conflict and the following consequences: communication used for negative purpose, lack of ability to express themselves, break in communication, uncontrollable speech and energy drain thru endless talking, stubborn silence.

CHALLENGE

If you find yourself in a relationship lacking in communication, all aspects of your relationship will suffer. Unexpressed feelings, desires, wishes and discontent will prevent you from letting go, opening up, and clearly projecting to the world who you are and what you want or need. Until this is mastered you will not be able to ascend further in your spiritual evolutionary process.

REMEDY

Be acutely and entirely honest and open in voicing your needs and desires, as well as dislikes and discontent. Make time for peaceful, kind and loving conversation, nurture each other's ability to speak honestly without fear of consequences. Avoid stubborn silence at all costs, and curb your reactive speech that may be hurtful. Self-reflect and review your individual discoveries. Explore mental and emotional communication on a telepathic level of higher awareness. If both partners are synchronized at this level, they will not experience any conflicts.

ASPECTS ~ Voice, truth, communication, higher knowledge
LOCATION ~Throat
COLOR ~ Blue
SENSE ~ Hearing

Speak from Your Heart:

"My words are my truth. You are the most important person to me."

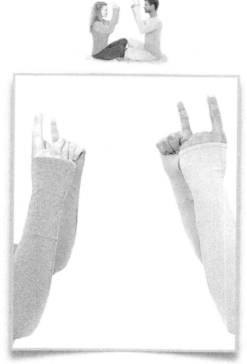

Sit with a straight back and face your partner, knees touching lightly. Lift the arms up, elbows at the shoulder level. Make fists with both hands, leaving thumbs on the outside. Now stretch both index fingers and point them towards the sky. Hold for three minutes. **Breath is long, deep and slow.** Gaze into each other's eyes and look deeply into the divinity within you. Project unconditional love and surrender to the feeling of complete oneness. Transcend all earthly desires and strive to become united in the finer frequency, activate your ability to ascend to the next level of consciousness.

Affirmation:

**WE LISTEN TO EACH OTHER AND SPEAK WORDS OF LOVE,
TRUTH AND LIGHT.**

MUDRA *for* CHAKRA 6.

DYNAMICS

If two souls vibrate at this high - energy frequency, they are in absolute alignment with their life purpose, mission and have the ability to sense and receive visions from far past, and future. This state promotes abilities of high perception, realization, and such a pairing of two souls inspires calmness and peace in others. At this level of spiritual evolvement there is no danger for spiritual reversal or descent.

WEAKNESS AND IMBALANCE

Disharmony and incompatibility in this chakra center can create conflict and the following consequences: incompatible disposition towards life in general, life purpose, and higher spiritual concepts as well as general priorities. If both partners are synchronized at this level, they will not experience any real conflicts.

CHALLENGE

If you find yourself in a relationship lacking in spiritual alignment, it will eventually affect other areas of your partnership. You will feel deeply disconnected and when physical attraction subsides the relationship will get distant and most likely fall apart. Until this level is mastered, you will not be able to ascend further in the final step of your spiritual evolutionary process.

REMEDY

Honest communication of your higher principles and intentions will help you lessen the distance between two partners that are not compatible on this level. You may remain in a partially satisfactory relationship, but will have to resign to the fact that your spiritual quest will not be something you will be able to share with your partner. This dynamic is possible if many other aspects are compatible, however it will never be as fulfilling. The less evolved partner will have to be at least at the fourth chakra level of ascension. If you have met your compatible partner that understands and compliments your true spiritual essence and functions on this - your frequency level, you are incredibly fortunate and blessed. Take this opportunity to ascend as high as possible thru unconditional love, and fluidly merge your mission for the highest purpose and the betterment of this world.

ASPECTS ~ Third Eye, vision, intuition
LOCATION ~Third Eye
COLOR ~ Indigo

Speak from Your Heart:
" We are One now and forever. We see beyond here and now."

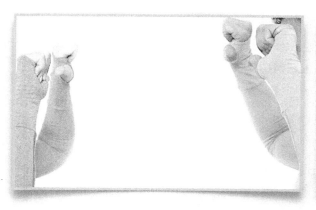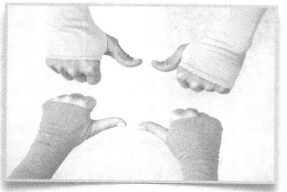

Sit with a straight back and face your partner, knees touching lightly. Lift the hands up to the level of your head, make fists with both hands leaving the thumbs outside. Point the stretched thumb tips against the side of your head between the eyebrows and your ears, not touching your head. Breathe and concentrate onto your partner's eyes, sending loving energy and devotion, while honoring your own inner truth. Practice for three minutes and see the divinity in your partner.

Breath is long, deep and slow. Look deeply into your partner's eyes, project unconditional love and remain in a meditative state, consciously lifting your focus upwards and visualizing energy from the bottom of your spine ascending up towards your third eye center. The thumbs send energy to your 6th Chakra, so the two of you together create an energy body of tremendous magnitude and attunement. With this strong joint energy body you have established, your energy is magnified and optimal for accomplishing enlightening tasks for the betterment of all.

Affirmation:
WE EMBRACE THE PAST, PRESENT AND THE FUTURE, AND KNOW OUR MISSION.

MUDRA for CHAKRA 7.

DYNAMICS

This is the final and optimal state of union of two souls before they return to their creator. All feelings, desires and emotions are dissolved as they remain in a state of pure bliss and joy.

WEAKNESS AND IMBALANCE

Disharmony and incompatibility in this chakra center can create conflict and the following consequences: incompatible state of existence. If both partners are synchronized at this level, they are completely united and function in perfect harmony and attract powerful synchronicity into every area of their life.

CHALLENGE

If you find yourself in a relationship where one partner is at this high level and the other partner isn't, they can function together but under unusual circumstances and in a very different relationship dynamic as expected. The more evolved partner is removed from daily life and exists in solitude and silence. The less evolved partner understands and accepts this dynamic and deals with earthly matters that need tending to. This is by no means an equal dynamic, but often an accepted one. The less evolved partner has to be at least at the fourth chakra level of ascension. Until this level is mastered you will not be able to ascend further to complete and finalize your spiritual evolutionary process on earth.

REMEDY

When two partners are not synchronized at this level, the relationship becomes a matter of personal choice, as is always anyway. Certainly the less evolved partner will most likely also be a highly evolved individual, who will understand this relationship from perhaps a heart centered unconditional love - level. This is a very unusual dynamic and does not happen often to say the least. If you are the less evolved partner, you consciously decide to remain in their relationship and learn. The evolved partner will not be able to include you in his experiences, therefore he will be the dominant one even by not exercising this position, it will be a matter of consequence to this set up. If both partners are at this level of ascension, they are highly evolved souls, who have an important purpose, mission and work to accomplish, with a very clear goal of helping the world and others. Every couple should strive to reach this level and be inspired by the possibility and clarity, that this is where their final journey is taking them. In state of complete unity with each other and the creator, the limitations of this dimension cease to exist and you have completed your sojourn here on earth.

ASPECTS ~ The Universal God consciousness, the heavens, unity, humility
LOCATION ~ Top of the head, crown
COLOR ~ Violet & white

Speak from Your Heart:

"We are blissful, connected to the eternal source.
We are limitless in our love for each other and our service to others".

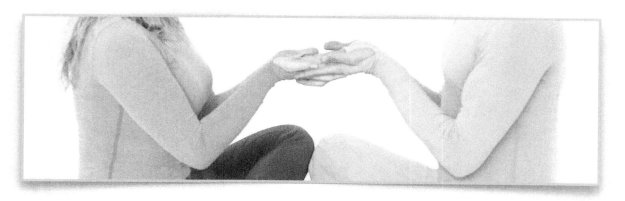

Sit with a straight back and face your partner, knees touching lightly. Lift the hands up to the level of your hearts, and hold the palms facing up, facing the sky. Now intertwine your fingers with your partner's, while the palms still face up. Feel the strong energy currents in your interlaced fingers and centers of palms.

Breathe long, deep and slow. Look deeply into your partner's eyes and see his true divinity and soul in its purest form. With each breath consciously visualize your energy currents lifting into your crown center, and opening your receptivity of the highest Universal power. Life force is streaming into your hands, entering your hearts, and ascending towards your crown. Remain in this state of purity and blissful merging for at least three minutes.

Affirmation:

WE ARE PURE BLISS, ONE WITH EACH OTHER
AND THE CREATOR.

Part Four

Heal Your Heart

*My heart is as vulnerable as a most delicate flower with its petals stretching towards the summer sky,
waiting for one tiny gentle raindrop. It has been a hot, dry summer and I am thirsty.
One fresh dewdrop is all I need and I will continue to bloom, share my mesmerizing scent
and fascinate you with my unusual beauty. I am that flower don't you see?
Please protect me with a gentle caress, so that I can share my beauty
and in gratitude feed your soul with my essence.*

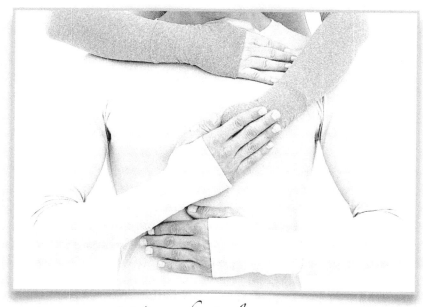

Mudra of Healing Hearts

Mudra for Overcoming Conflict

Whenever two mighty forces meet, energy currents connect, merge and in this moment of adjustments it is natural that clashes occur. They bring up old wounds, fears and insecurities. Instead of running away, remaining silent or pretending a dark cloud doesn't exist, gather your courage to stand in front of each other, naked with vulnerability and allow the thunderstorm to wash you clean. Now you can exhale and smile again, because you have seen each other in the weakest moment, without defenses, walls, or veils of lies. You know your beautiful invisible entity of love and where it is vulnerable or weak, and together you can help heal and move beyond the experiences past. With wisdom gained and confidence that you will never go down the old path again, you are creating your new paradise and nobody can touch it.

This Mudra set will help you feel your partner's love thru the back - the easier path to heart center. You have each other's back and there is nothing to fear, you are safe.

Speak from Your Heart:

I have traveled thru my life, and had my heart broken,
and each time I picked up the million little pieces and bravely moved on.
I love myself enough to dare to love again.
Now that I found you, my heart opened once more.
I can't pretend to you that I am always fearless.
I trust you with the sorrow of my past, I know you can help me
heal my vulnerable secret compartments and teach me once again
how to love without fear, tears or compromising my heart's ability to love unconditionally.
I trust that you are the one who will cherish and protect my love,
because this is the last time my heart is this beautiful and open.
It is you or nobody else. Can you stand strong?

Affirmation:
WE ARE ONE.
WE LOVE, TRUST AND PROTECT EACH OTHER.

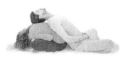 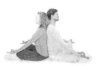 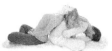

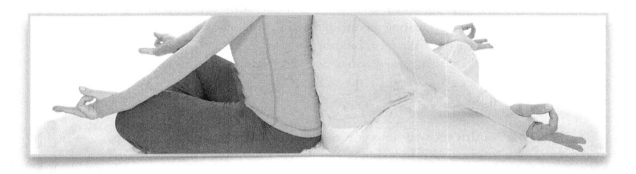

Sit back to back with a straight spine. Take a deep breath, exhale and bend forward with your partner leaning back onto you, relaxing with his full weight on your back. Remain for a few moments and then inhale while extending your body upwards and leaning back onto your partners back. Open your heart and relax for a few moments and then repeat the movement forward. Repeat and continue for three minutes. Now place your hands on your knees, stretch your fingers, connect the thumbs and index fingers forming a circle, both palms facing up towards the sky. There are two options for finger position: you can connect precisely the fingertips OR place the index fingers at the root of the thumb fingers. Hold for three minutes. Gaze into the distance or close your eyes and feel your hearts connecting through your back. This is an easier way to access the heart center - with less obstruction from the third - ego center, where conflicts occur. You are healing and reconnecting your hearts, while pushing ego out of the way. Project unconditional love.

Breath:

Long, deep and slow.

Mudra for Releasing Control

The issue of control in a relationship is very often a challenge. But it takes two to play that game and as always it all begins with each partner individually, for if there is no weaker needy one, the other won't respond to that with the urge to control. When you let go of fear and realize that not everything in life can be controlled, you understand that it is only your ego that requires to be controlled, so it doesn't make a useless mess of all things beautiful. If you are too lazy to make choices and decisions, and expect someone else to make them for you, you are creating a control dynamic, pulling your partner into filling your missing ability with their own strength. Likewise, pay attention if you want to control others and why? It is a thankless fear based habit, one that has no place in an equal and evolved partnership. Tame it, let go, allow the Universe to play its song, and you'll be free.

**This Mudra set will help you release control in any relationship,
and balance the power equally.**

Speak from Your Heart:
*While we dance together the dance of life I'd like you to know,
you can sweep me off my feet and carry me, if you so feel.
I know that if I ask, you will place me gently on the ground again, and I'll be free to dance as I want.
I'd like you to know that I will do the same for you.
So there is no need for control, because my spirit is free and uncatchable, as is yours.
But my soul longs to dance in a pair, and I love a mate who also knows how to lead.
In a perfect dance, each partner carries their strength equally, and together their souls sing with the universe.*

Affirmation:
**WE ARE EQUAL, RELEASING CONTROL
AND BREATHING AS ONE.**

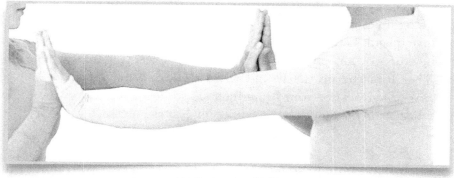

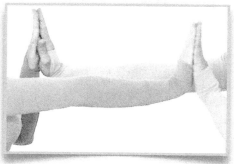

Sit facing your partner, keep the back nice and straight, long neck, shoulders down. Your knees are almost touching. Lift the hands up to heart level, both palms facing your partner. Now place both hands together palm to palm with your partner's, your right with his left and your left with his right hand. Inhale and stretch the right hand forward, while simultaneously bending the left at the elbow. Next, while exhaling bend the right elbow while stretching the left one. Repeat for three minutes while looking deeply into your partner's eyes. Your right hand is your mental side, while the left one your emotional side. With each inhalation and movement of the right hand, you are relaxing the mental "grip", while your left hand helps you both to balance your emotions connected to issues of control. Look into your partner's eyes with love and openness to release all control and merge as one harmonious entity. Project unconditional love.

Breath:

Long, deep and slow.

Mudra for Diminishing Insecurities

Insecurity stems from feeling fearful and doubting in your own abilities. Past hurts can contribute to these self-doubts and create a feeling of unworthiness that permeates your actions, decisions and choices in partnerships. When you attract an equal partner, they too may be healing insecurities from their past, and together you can reassure as well as remind each other how special you are, how pure your intentions are, and how able and deserving you are of the most fulfilling and beautiful love relationship. An equal pairing will magnify your own positive qualities and bring you more power, strength and confirmation that as a result of staying true to your self, and your higher principles, you are now precisely where you selected. Therefore choose wisely and when needed, remind yourself of your self-worth and help your partner see your beautiful soul, so deserving and giving of love. And reassure each other, that you are perfect and enough, just as you are.

This Mudra helps you remain strong in character, empowers your inner integrity, reminding you of the natural sense of security from within.

Speak from Your Heart:

In today's world I feel vulnerable in my expected attributes and abilities.
The pressure for perfection surrounds me everyday and I have to work continuously
to keep my inner balance, and self - awareness while staying true to myself.
I hold my own power, but still my partner is my rock, my mirror,
reminding me that we both need each other
to keep the balance while wild ocean waves of life keep tossing us around our relationship.
There are only the two of us onboard and together we will overcome anything, for we are unbeatable.
But I may ask you sometimes if you are still on board with me, so just say "Yes", that's all I need.
I know you are, but I like hearing your voice telling me so.

Affirmation:

WE FEEL CONFIDENT IN THE
INDESTRUCTIBLE POWER OF OUR LOVE.

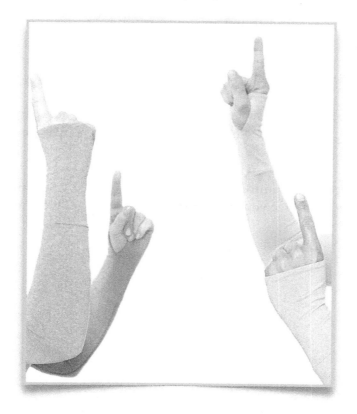

Mudra for a Strong Character is practiced sitting with a straight back, while facing your partner. Next, extend index fingers while bending the rest, thumb crossing over. Now lift the hands, right one at the height of your forehead, left one at the height of your shoulder. Stretch the index fingers and point them towards the sky. Breathe while gazing lovingly into your partner's eyes, sending loving energy and devotion, while honoring your own inner truth. Practice for three minutes and see the divinity in your partner.

Breath:

Long, deep and slow.

Mudra for Eliminating Possessiveness

When the flames of passion take over, there are many other emotional nuances that appear, waiting to take part in this magnetic interaction. The energy between two people is so hypnotizing that you need to understand and know yourself as well as your own reactions to this overwhelming emotional exchange. You may feel out of control and so intertwined with your mate that naturally fear appears without a warning. Fear of losing your love can manifest in the form of sudden unexpected possessiveness, which will only make your partner feel unhappy and trapped, and that will only prompt him to want to leave these energy restrictions. Let go and know he will only be with you if he wants to, and not if you allow possessiveness to take over, and change you into something that you're not.

This Mudra will help you tranquilize your mind, strengthen your bond with calmness and confidence, and give you the ability to overcome all weakness and fear.

Speak from Your Heart:

I know that your presence is a gift to me and you will only stay if you feel loved and understood.
I sense your need to feel the wind in your hair without restrictions
while you run like a wild horse through the prairie.
But I also know that I am yours and you will remain loyal and always come back because your heart is
with me, and that's enough for me. If you see me tremble with fear of losing you and see that even a hint
of possessiveness is trying to take me hostage, understand that I don't like it, and don't want it.
Instead of scolding me and forcing me to defend myself, just embrace me with a smile
and it will all evaporate into thin air in an instant.

Affirmation:
WE BELONG TO THE UNIVERSE.

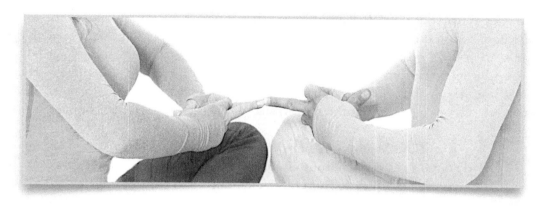

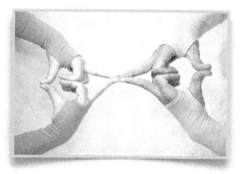

With this Mudra for Tranquilizing the Mind, you need to sit with a straight back and face your partner, your knees almost touching with his. Now connect the middle fingertips and point them away from your body. Bend the rest of the fingers, connect the thumb tips and point them towards your solar plexus, the rest of the fingers are bent and touching back to back at the middle knuckles till fingertips. Now connect your touching middle fingertips with your partner's middle fingertips and feel the instant powerful energy flow between you. This Mudra will help your tranquilize the mind and overcome restless and negative feelings of possessiveness. Breathe and keep looking into your partner's eyes with love, confidence and utmost peace. Send him love and see deeply into his soul. You have nothing to fear, let go and be in the moment. Practice for three minutes.

Breath:

Long, deep and slow.

Mudra for Conquering Obstacles

Life is full of obstacles, but the difference is how you see them. Do you understand the hidden messages within them, do you respect the time they demand, the explorations and creativity they push you into? Perhaps the seeming obstacles are really helpers so you may select the best option on how to proceed, or really understand how important something or someone is to you. If everything is easy, you may dismiss its value. If something takes an effort, you will understand its importance. And then? The obstacles will disappear, because you passed the lesson they offered. When two people love each other in a most elevated expression, no obstacle will prevent them from sharing their love, for it will conquer all.

**The Mudra will help you develop patience
and remain reflective about challenges and wise with choices.
The connected middle fingers will synchronize your strengths.**

Speak from Your Heart:

*I know what I want and when the gravitation of Earth seemingly delays fulfilling my wishes,
I study myself and see how important you are to me.
I become more acutely aware of time and the power of thoughts,
and I cherish every second we have together even more, because each one is a most precious gift.
So the obstacles make me love you even more.*

Affirmation:

**TOGETHER WE WILL CONQUER ANYTHING,
WE WORK WITH THE PERFECT TIMING OF THE UNIVERSE.**

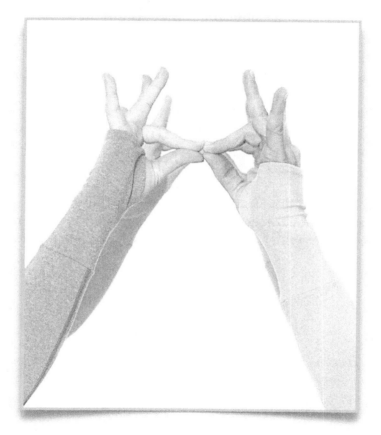

Sit with a straight back facing your partner, knees are almost touching. Connect the middle and thumb fingertips stretching out the rest of the fingers. Now turn your palms towards your partner and place the two connected fingertips of your hands – your middle and thumb fingertips -together with your partner's. Patiently look into each other's eyes and project unconditional love, loyalty and strength. Practice for three minutes.

Breath:

Long, deep and slow.

Mudra for Dismissing Outside Influences

When two equals meet in love, their light is blinding and many can not bear its power. They may fight against you, using all their might to plant seeds of doubt or darkness all around you. However, by remaining strong and resilient, you will overcome these outside forces and prevail in your strength with pure intentions for the higher good. Your true love is a force to be reckoned with and your higher mission must and will be accomplished. It is essential to understand who you are together, and never doubt it for a second, just hold the light, surround each other with love and consciously magnify it. The universe will help you. Why? Because the two of you are the Agents of Light and the Universe works thru you.

**This Mudra of ancient Egypt will protect you
from any outside forces that may not be in your best interest.
It creates an energy field of perfect inner balance and outer shield.**

Speak from Your Heart:

*I know that no matter what surrounds us, you will always hold my hand and guard my back.
And you must know that I will be your fierce protector till my last breath in this world.
Nothing will break us apart and no one can touch us. Together we are invincible.
Never doubt that, and in return I will neither.*

Affirmation:

**WE ARE UNBEATABLE,
UNWAVERING IN OUR LOVE FOR EACH OTHER.**

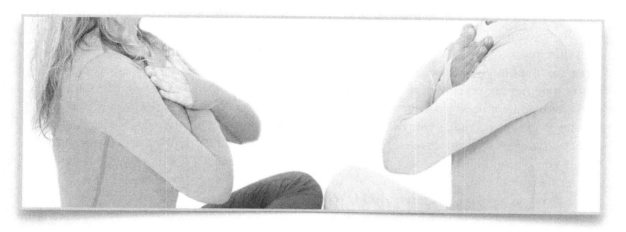

Sit with a straight back facing your partner, your knees touching lightly. Place your right hand over your heart, palm on your chest. And now place the left hand over the right, palm on the right side of your chest, both hands are at same height. Look into your partner's eyes and remain closely connected, creating your own energy field that is impenetrable to all outside stimuli. This is your protected joint energy body, maintained by your dedicated love. Breathe and gaze into each other's eyes and project pure unconditional love. See the divine in your partner and expand your perception, consciously projecting a large field of protective light all around you. Hold it in your minds together, and feel it permeate every cell of your combined energy body. You always carry a protective shield, but when you consciously activate it, its power is magnified unimaginably so. Practice for three minutes.

Breath:

Long, deep and slow.

Mudra for Evoking Happiness

Happiness is one of the most powerful and healthy supremely necessary healer. It doesn't have to be complicated and it doesn't take much. You can be happy doing very little, perhaps observing nature, letting yourself go, and surrendering to the moment. No tools are needed, only your willing awareness.What's important is your ability to recognize true happiness and never take it for granted. Most often we remember happiness more than actually recognize it in the moment. By reminding each other how very special and blissful each minute of joy is, we etch it in eternity and keep it in our hearts forever. This way it can serve us indefinitely, and continuously infuse us with its power and energy. Two happy hearts together are certainly even more powerful than one, but the key is to understand and cultivate true happiness on your own and never weigh it down with expectations that your partner is going to "make you happy". When you're able to be happy on your own, you'll attract a likewise soul into your life and together your happiness will exceed expectations. When you encounter a time of challenge, remind each other of your happiest moments and let them fuel your strenuous journey to the next supremely happy occasion. Happiness needs to be recognized, appreciated and cultivated.

**This Mudra will help you establish, maintain and strengthen
a genuine sense of happiness and inner joy.**

Speak from Your Heart:

*My heart longs to be happy and share each magnificent moment of love with you.
I know that by joining our heart's celebration, we magnify our power and spread it to others. If we encounter a moment of weakness, and don't recognize the true blessing of happiness all around us, let's kindly remind each other and return back where we began…with a welcome smile, a gentle caress and a happiness infused open heart.*

Affirmation:
**I OPEN MY HEART TO JOY AND CHERISH EACH MOMENT
OF HAPPINESS WITH YOU.**

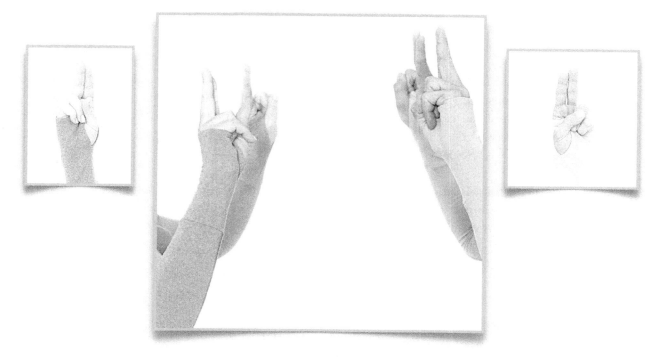

Sit with a straight back facing your partner, your knees touching lightly. Lift both hands up, elbows slightly below shoulder level. Turn the open palms towards your partner, extend the index and middle fingers and bend the ring and little fingers, the thumbs are crossing over the two bent fingers. This Mudra for happiness will help you establish a sense of inner joy and higher vibration.

Breathe long, deep and slow. Project pure joy, happiness and love to each other. Look deeply into each other's eyes and see the purely divine spirit. Practice for three minutes.

Breath:

Long, deep and slow.

Mudra for Overcoming Societal Restrictions

Being one of a kind and different sounds exciting, but it has its price. You are a trailblazer, breaking the rules, expectations and this very often frightens people. Everything people don't know they are usually afraid of, or quick to judge. So you have to know that if your relationship is in any way different then the expected norm, you are an example teaching others to expand their horizons and eliminate judgments. When two people fall in love and are faced with societal restrictions in any kind of way, this presents a test of their love. But quite often if their love is strong and true, the obstacle will bring them even closer, for they recognize that love truly conquers all and has no boundaries. Love is the greatest power of the Universe and transcends the limitations of time, space or even death. Societal restrictions that are in any way wanting to control your love are meaningless and powerless, for true love is indestructible.

This Mudra of strength will help you join your power to overcome any outside restrictive and limiting influences. Your energy field of love is impenetrable and protected.

Speak from Your Heart:

In so many unspoken words society has certain expectations of you and I.
If I am different and live my life on my unique schedule,
and love whom my heart chooses, that is my birthright.
I love you regardless of the earthly expectations, I love you for your timeless essence
and nothing, no person, or manmade restriction will ever change that.
And if the whole world disappears, I will still love you, forever.

Affirmation:
**YOU ARE THE ANCHOR OF MY HEART,
THE SAFE HAVEN FOR MY SOUL.**

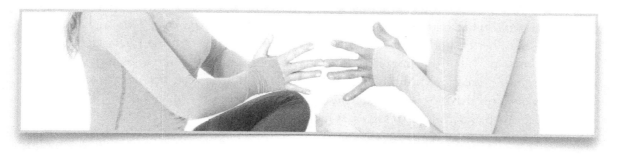

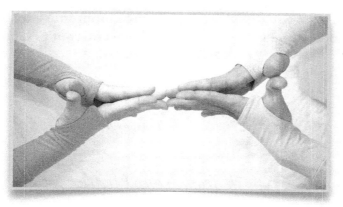

Sit with a straight back facing your partner, knees almost touching. Press your hands together, palms touching and fingers stretched and spread apart. Hold the hands in front of your solar plexus area, thumbs pointing up towards the sky. Now join your middle touching fingertips with your partner's and hold, breathing as one, long, deep and slow. Feel the powerful energy current connecting thru your middle fingertips and moving into and throughout your body. The energy in your pressed palms and connected middle fingers creates an energy current magnifier that you will sense in your heart and throughout your body. The combined strength of the two of you, charges your energy circuits. Look into your partner's eyes with love and complete openness, in awareness that the two of you have the joined strength to overcome any obstacle that comes your way. Project unconditional love and hold for three minutes.

Breath:

Long, deep and slow.

Mudra for Finding Compromise

The mastery of finding compromise in a relationship is something worth developing no matter how set you are in your habits. Instead of seeing this as a sacrifice, or having to change or adapt certain aspects of yourself, see it really for what it truly is: an incredible opportunity to expand your horizons and attempt to see the world from a different perspective. And what better perspective then that of your loved one. This way you will know him even better, understand him deeper, and love him even more. Every element of your relationship will grow in this ability and your bond will intertwine into such an intricate beautiful creation, nobody else will be able to touch. That becomes your unique love experience on the most essential level of human existence - of living this human life through your own and your lover's eyes. What a treasure to behold.

This Mudra set helps you develop the ability to compromise with your partner by balancing and harmonizing both sides of your personality, the mind and the heart.

Speak from Your Heart:

*I want to know you, and every tiny detail about you. And I wish you are as curious about me.
Understanding your opinions or wishes that are different or even opposite of mine,
will help me experience life from your place, through your eyes, ears and your senses.
I will understand what makes your heart beat faster and what makes your soul sing.
I want to know that, and I would not call that a compromise.
I would call it an expansion of my awareness, a most precious lover's gift.*

Affirmation:
**WITH LOVE I CAN SEE, FEEL AND UNDERSTAND
THE WORLD THRU YOUR EYES.**

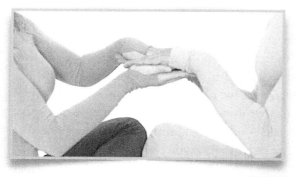
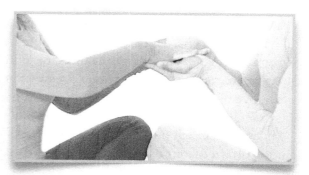

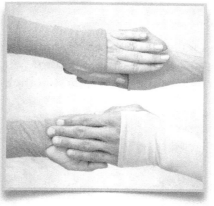

Sit with a straight back, facing your partner, your knees are touching lightly. Lift up your hands at chest level and hold the left hand palm facing up all fingers together and right hand facing down, all fingers together. Now place the right hand on top of your partner's upturned left palm and your upturned left hand is offering a safe place for rest for your partner's right hand. This mudra helps you balance the mind, mental, and ego side of your relationship. Breathe long deep and slow and hold for three minutes, gazing into your partner's eyes and opening your energy to feel mutual love. Now reverse the position of the hands, your right palm facing up towards the sky holding your partner's left hand and your left facing down and resting on your partner's upturned right hand. Breathe long, deep and slow and hold for three minutes. This Mudra helps you nurture and harmonize the emotional side of your relationship. Gaze into your partner's eyes and willingly open your heart and mind to blending and working as one, in complete loving harmony and balance. Project unconditional love and understanding. Upon gazing into his eyes with love, see your own reflection.

Breath:

Long, deep and slow.

Mudra for Transcending Patterns

Until we met each other we each lived and traveled thru life in a certain way. Once we were blessed with our love, everything changed in an instant. Now our world is not the same, our laughter is filled with sparkles of pure light and our tears are caressed away by each others loving hand. The dance tempo has shifted, the sunsets are richer and the beauty of life magnified. And yes, everything was beautiful before, but now that we are reunited, the pattern has changed. We created a new pattern from the moment we met. And if during our love dance we may feel stuck in an old boring song, we can change the music and dance differently. All it takes is our clear connection and awareness of where the music takes us, while we feel each other's inner rhythm. Let's be still for a magical moment that will reveal a new pattern of our dance, so together, we may dance to the heavens.

**This Mudra will release pent up energy and open up
your creative inner awareness so that you may find a clear direction
of your next journey together.**

Speak from Your Heart:

*Yes, I know we want everything to stay perfect just as it is in this sublime moment.
But have no fear of moving forward into our next moment in life,
where things may seem and will be different than now.
It will still be the two of us, no matter what happens or where we land.
Just remember, I will be at your side, catching up or guiding you,
so we shall never lose sight of each other.*

Affirmation:
**WE ARE FEARLESS IN CHANGING
AND DISCOVERING OUR FUTURE.**

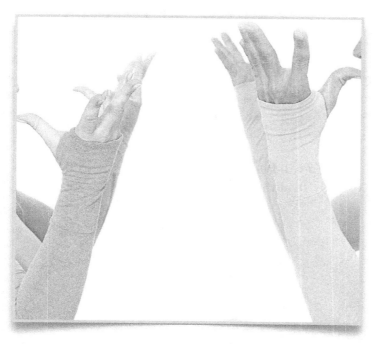

Sit with a straight back, facing your partner and lightly touching each other's knees. Lift your hands up to face level, elbows comfortably to the sides, away from your body and palms open as if holding a ball. All fingers are stretched and pointing up towards the sky. Now begin twirling your hands at the wrists, inwards and outwards at a fast pace. Breathe and continue for three minutes. This mudra is quite a challenge in persistence and stamina, but lovingly and with determination connect with your partner and merge your sheer will power and persistence so that you may overcome your weaker moments. Keep the elbows nice and high and do not give up. Continue on for three minutes. Look into each other's eyes and help sustain mutual strength. Persist and you will experience powerful energy shifts. Continue to look deeply and lovingly into each other's eyes, and with determination and focus help break the old and create a new incarnation of the winning team - the two of you.

Breath:

Long, deep and slow.

Mudra for Forgiveness and Letting Go

We all carry a certain amount of "space" within our mindset, heart capacity and emotional memories. It is important to be very selective about what you hold in your memory bank and weed out the things that don't serve your best interests. In every relationship endless adventures happen, as do misunderstandings and moments of fear or hurt. It is truly all about our ability to communicate clearly with each other, and take enough time to simply understand what your partner needs, wants and also what makes them fearful. Letting go of all unnecessary emotional baggage is essential, so that you create space for positive, empowering and most loving dynamics that you can infuse into everything you create, touch and experience together. Consciously learn to let go of the old and make space for wonderful new experiences.

**This Mudra will help you find forgiveness and harmony
so that you may heal the past, and open the gates of your future.**

Speak from Your Heart:

*I tell you what frightens me, I know you will help me blow away my fears.
If I tell you when your words strike me in my most vulnerable delicate tissue,
I know you will make sure to not wound me again. And I can let go and trust you completely,
because I know you want me to be free to enjoy our bliss, just like I want the same for you.
Let's release everything we don't want or need, so it is just the two of us,
alone in the beautiful oasis of our love and life.*

Affirmation:
**WE HEAL AND LEAVE THE PAST BEHIND
AND SAIL FORWARD WITH GLORY IN OUR EYES.**

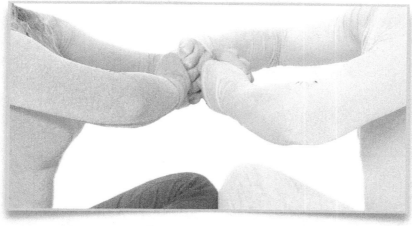

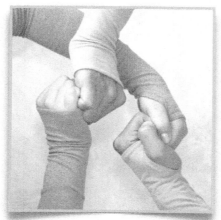

Sit with a straight back facing your partner, your knees touching lightly. Lift the hands up to the level of your heart, interconnect your hands by hooking them in a lightly open fist, your right palm looking towards your partner- your left palm turned inward, towards your heart. Breathe and practice for three minutes. Gaze into your partner's eyes with open heart, unconditional love and compassion. Feel the love pouring into each other thru the direct connection of hands, and observe a sense of deep peace and harmony that envelops you both.

Breath:

Long, deep and slow.

Part Five

Purify Your Mind

*Make no mistake, your mind plays a crucial role in when, how and under what restrictions
your heart receives an opportunity to love. When your mind gets out of the way or even helps the heart to emerge,
your soul sings with joy, for finally your true essence comes forth and you are precisely who you are supposed to be —
a carefree spirit filled with abundance of joy, laughter and love.
When the heart tames the mind, your true nature blossoms.*

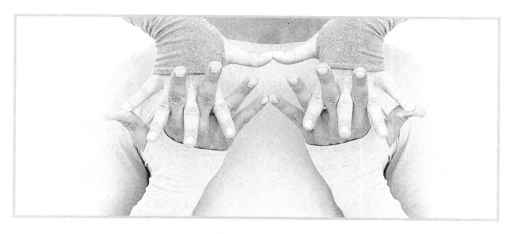

Mudra of Mental Synchronicity

Mudra for Activating Love

Love needs all the perfect conditions to thrive and breathe within our hearts. It needs a proper mindset, attention, time, clear and open dialogue pathways, empty of negativity and ready to give as well as receive. When our daily lives continuously take us away into the chaos of the crowd, we need to consciously return to our hearts. Together, create the most important sacred space where your love can reignite and thrive. And each time upon your return into your guarded place of light, call on your love, with clear intention and fearless open heart. It will hear your call and eagerly return from the depths of your soul, to help you remember why you're alive.

This Mudra will help you quiet your mind and open your heart,
while activating the clear energy pathways of your little fingers,
the main channels of communication.

Speak from Your Heart:
All I want is you next to me and nothing else.
And we can be quiet and completely still and our world will be perfect.
I have this longing in my heart, to belong and just be. To feel protected and loved in your arms.
And only then in such a perfect moment, I am able to feel safe enough to completely surrender
and open my heart like a flower, trusting while waiting for the morning sun.
Nothing else exists, only you and I, in our blissful stillness of love.
I am here with my heart open, now and forever…only for you.

Affirmation:
I SURRENDER MY HEART AND
TRUST IN OUR BREATH AS ONE.

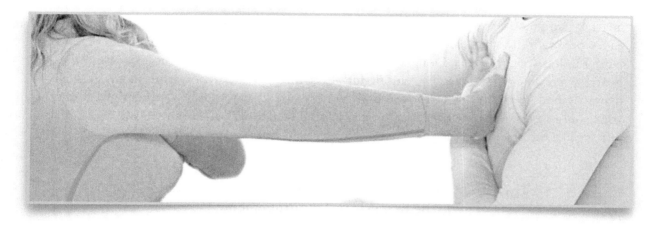

Sit with a straight spine, facing your partner, your knees touching lightly. Place your right hand on your partner's heart, and your left hand on the right side of your chest. Breathe while gazing into each other's eyes. Feel the soothing energy of your partner's palm on your heart. Hold for three minutes. See his divinity. Practice for three minutes and project unconditional love.

Breath:

Long, deep and slow.

Mudra for Better Communication

Communication is everything. And the beautiful thing about a love relationship is that you can communicate in so many ways, and on so many levels that are not restricted to just verbal exchange. You can alter your lives with one deep look into each other's eyes, a gentle sigh into his ear, a soft but electric touch, or while leaving behind a seductive trace of your scent. This kind of communication is instantaneous in triggering sensory responses and actually not a single spoken word is necessary. How about communicating when you are far apart, when you don't have the luxury of standing next to each other? Well, then there are those otherworldly skills that two highly attuned souls possess, and you can further develop with Mudras. Such skills as long distance communication of strong thought projection, heart synchronicity, and parallel emotional attunement create a powerful and irresistible magnetic pull. If you try to resist, you only end up miserable because you can't fight against your soul's resonance with a soulmate or twin soul. That kind of communication is a real gift, it's like the Sun…it is there, everyday in every way, and you need it for life.

**This Mudra set will help you elevate your communication
to the highest level of attunement.**

Speak from Your Heart:

Our communication is everything to me.
When days are long and nights are cold, your words are like a fire that keeps my heart alive.
And when life overwhelms me, you are the fresh exotic drink
that sends a vibrant remedy throughout my body.
Your silence confuses and devastates me, but you reaching out to me even in most invisible but loving ways,
sends me into an exalted state of knowing that you are with me, always singing to my soul.
I can listen to you endlessly and know you will do the same for me.
Remember, our pure love needs that, so it can live forever.

Affirmation:
**I LISTEN AND HEAR YOU
WITH MY OPEN AND LOVING HEART.**

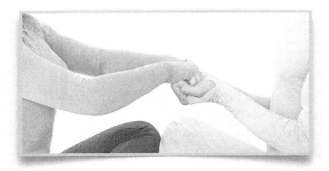
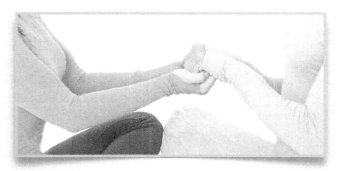

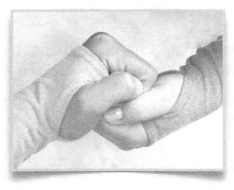

Sit with a straight back, facing your partner and knees touching lightly. Lift your hands to heart level and softly form open fists with both hands, palms facing down. Your partner will form soft open fists with palms facing up, towards the sky. Now you will hook your hands together, him holding your palms safely in his hands. Breathe and gaze into each other's eyes. This is a Mudra for non-verbal communication with him listening to you. Hold for three minutes and tell him with your eyes how you feel about him and how much you love him. Now reverse the position and hold his hands in the safety of your upturned hands hooking and fitting nicely together creating a feeling of coziness and comfort. Breathe and gaze into each other's eyes, with him conveying to you his feelings by unspoken words of love frequency. Hold for three minutes and project unconditional love towards each other.

Breath:

Long, deep and slow.

Mudra for Deepening Physical Connection

When two lovers step into the endless ocean of love, many beautiful events take place. One of them, the physical merging, becomes another way of experiencing closeness. It is, in fact, the closest you can get to each other in this limited three-dimensional world. To make that experience something entirely different and so much more than the limited physical blending, you can expand your hearts with unconditional love and merge with your highest consciousness, so that your physical love elevates into a true melting of two souls. This magical experience transcends all others and has the potential to catapult you into stratosphere of unconditional cosmic love and ecstasy. For that to occur, both of you need three essential non-negotiable ingredients: a pure and open heart, an expanded and fine tuned ability of the mind, and deep unconditional love for each other. This miraculous ascension requires two absolutely equal participants. This way, together, you may enter a different, exquisitely ethereal world.

**This Mudra set will help you feel,
sense and merge with each other's finer, ethereal body.**

Speak from Your Heart:

*You need to know that by opening my sacred gates to you, they offer more than just a temporary visit,
for you will turn into a permanent presence within my temple. From that moment on,
I will carry your essence around with me and breathe, cry, laugh and love with you wherever I go.
If you surrender, we will be free, if you hesitate and hold back, I will be wounded.
The gate to my temple and heart is open wide, but only for you.
Take a breath before you enter,
for it may be your last of this limited earthly dimension.*

Affirmation:
I SURRENDER TO THE DIVINE LOVE IN YOU, I AM YOU.

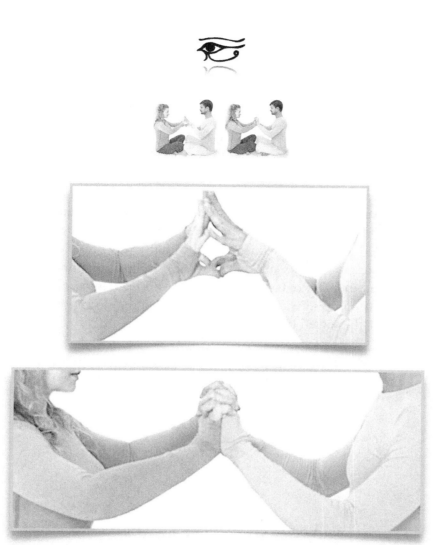

Sit with a straight back facing each other, knees lightly touching. Lift your hands to heart level, and turn the palms towards your partner, connect all the fingertips to his, while your outstretched fingers are held wide apart. Breathe and hold for three minutes. Look into your partner's eyes and feel the powerful interaction and blending of joined energy currents. Now keep the hands at the same level, and simply interlace the fingers clasping them together, palm to palm, fingers tightly intertwined. Breathe and practice for three minutes. Send loving energy into your partner's eyes, while looking deeply into his soul. Connect on the deepest level possible, feeling the energy force between palms, hold your joint frequency with ascending intention. Feel the divine in each other and see your reflection in his eyes. You are One.

Breath:

Long, deep and slow.

Mudra for Establishing Harmony

The key to maintaining unbreakable harmony within a partnership is to first conquer unrest within your own being. Most often when one partner is off balance, their partner is likewise susceptible to being affected, and the entire delicate equilibrium is thrown off. Both partners can be vulnerable and outside events can throw us off track, but being a team offers you a great advantage in conquering this challenge. In a moment of your partner's weakness, stand up and remain the anchor for you both. Your power will hold steady and maintain your essential harmonious frequency, and within a short time your partner's being will return to resonate with yours. And if you are the one fighting a wave of life's challenges, he will be your pillar of strength to guide you back into your safe haven. This way you are unbeatable and resilient to anything that comes your way, connected eternally, two loyal protectors of the sacred love you have created.

**This Mudra set will help you cultivate,
deepen and maintain harmony at all times.**

Speak from Your Heart:

*My love for you is so pure and stretches way beyond the horizon.
No matter what darkness throws at us, I will always hold our light in my heart
and the flame won't even tremble in midst of most furious winds. I will fight off anyone or anything
that tries to invade our sacred space, and guard our supreme peace and harmony with all my might.
No matter where we travel or live, our happiness and peace is my oasis, my true home.*

Affirmation:
**OUR PEACE HAS ONLY ONE HOME -
IN OUR LOVING HEARTS.**

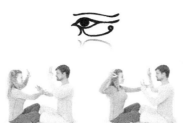

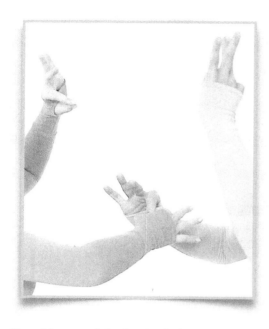
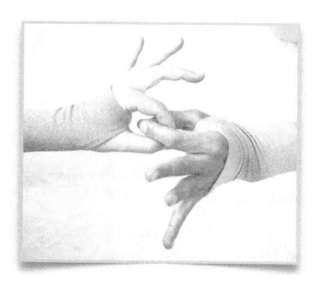

Sit with a straight back, facing your partner, knees touching lightly. Lift your right hand in front of your heart and connect the index and thumb fingertips. Stretch the rest of the fingers apart. Now interlock index and thumb fingers of your right hand with your partner's, forming a "Mudra chain" with two circles. Lift your left hand up, elbow at shoulder level and away from the body. Connect the index and thumb fingertips, all other fingers are spread out and stretched. Palm is facing away from your body, towards your partner. Breathe and hold for three minutes. Gaze into your partner's eyes and project love and mindful harmony. This part of the Mudra-set connects you on the deepest level of the mind. **Now reverse the position** and interlock the left hand fingers in the same Mudra, while holding the right hand up and away from your body. Breathe and again hold for three minutes. This part of the Mudra-set establishes complete harmony of the heart. Look into each other's eyes with deep love and compassion for each other, while you strengthen your invisible everlasting bond. Project love, peace, acceptance and harmony.

Breath:

Long, deep and slow.

Mudra for Yin Yang Balance

While we may look different, feel different and experience life differently when living as a man or a woman, we are tightly interconnected as well as interdependent. In fact, we complement each other and excel when blended together in a most magical combination.

 And each and every creation that we produce needs the perfect balance of these two of our essential energies. If we steer off course, or get lost in one direction, the other counterpart will suffer in neglect. Our relationship needs to respect and accommodate these essences we each carry in our individual unique combinations. As partners we attract that perfect missing blend that fits and completes ours. This fusion does not reduce our power, quite to the contrary, it makes it shine, it supports it and helps it express and manifest in its most beautiful form. We are like two perfect halves finally finding our way back to each other, so we can again vibrate at that sacred level where all differences cease to exits and we are one with the divine.

This Mudra evokes the manifestation of ideal,
finely delicate blend of your two energy poles.

Speak from Your Heart:

Where my body curves, you envelop it perfectly, because we were made for each other.
Where my mind travels, you meet me half way in the invisible field of endless dimensions.
When my heart sings, yours sings with me in a most lovely duet. Where my soul longs to return,
yours awaits at the sacred gates, so that together we create perfection and cease to exist in this limited world.
We become one with the universe, breathing with the ocean and shining with the sun.
You are my other half and together we are supreme.

Affirmation:
I HAVE THE SACRED COMBINATION YOU WANT
AND YOU HAVE MINE.

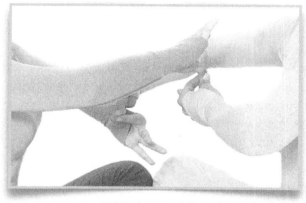

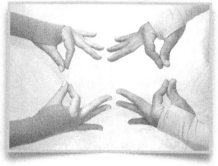

Sit with a straight back facing your partner, your knees touching lightly. With both hands, connect the index and thumb fingertips, all other fingers are stretched and spread out. Connect the tips of your connected right hand index and thumbs with the same tips of your partner's left hand, right palm facing out towards your partner. The index and thumb fingertips of your left hand are connected with the same tips of your partners right hand, your palm facing inward, towards you. Elbows are away from the body at the shoulder level. Breathe while looking deeply into your partner's eyes and seeing the pure divinity and beauty of his spirit. Hold for three minutes. This Mudra creates a perfect Yin Yang balance and is practiced always with the right hand (male side of one's nature) in the upper placement, while the female left hand (female side of one's nature) remains in lower placement, protected and receiving. Any couple combination (different or same sex) will strengthen their Yin Yang balance of these two power polarities, to best embellish and suit their individual needs.

Breath:

Long, deep and slow.

Mudra for Overcoming Stagnation

If time is an illusion, why worry about it needlessly? If change is a constant, why fight it uselessly? If standstill is always temporary, why not enjoy it and take advantage of feeling stationary? Every relationship experiences the inevitable and yet deceiving feeling of stagnation. There is no such thing, since everything is continuously moving, evolving, merging and traveling. As are the two of you. In such a special time, perhaps you can recognize the value of just being still, breathing and observing each other closely, remembering how many details your partner has that are so very attractive to you, those special secret signs you recognized when destiny presented you with this amazing gift of finding each other. If your every day is filled with ceaseless running, you can't see him, but in a moment of stillness you can truly lose yourself in him anew, deeply and with an open heart, like you did that very first time, when he appeared and took your breath away.

This Mudra will help you discover new creative ways of loving interaction.

Speak from Your Heart:

I promise that even if I see you every day, I won't forget your extraordinary loving heart.
I will look deeply into your eyes and find new nuances of you that make my heart tremble with delight.
And I invite you to listen to my heart and hear its fleeting ache for you,
the gentle whisper of its longing to remain in perfect concert with yours.
And every morning when I count my blessings that you are with me one more day,
open your eyes and remember, how blessed we are to have found each other, once again.

Affirmation:

**I SEE A BEAUTIFUL NEW MESSAGE FOR ME IN YOUR EYES,
EACH AND EVERY DAY.**

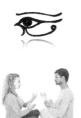

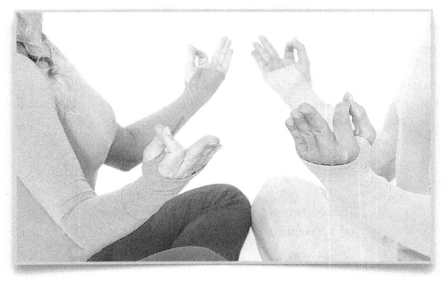

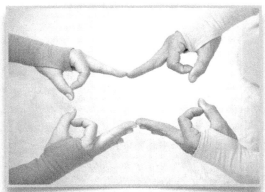

Sit with a straight back and face your partner, knees touching lightly. Lift your hands to the heart level, connect the index and thumb fingertips and stretch the rest of the fingers while holding them together, not separating. The palms are facing up towards the sky. Breathe and gaze into each other's eyes with new discovery in your intention. See the beauty and divine spirit in each other and project unconditional love. Practice for three minutes.

Breath:

Long, deep and slow.

Mudra for Sustaining Long Distance Love

When you find your true love, it doesn't matter where he is. It doesn't matter that you might not see him for a while, and it doesn't matter that you will miss him. All you care about, is that you found each other. In that moment of deep soul recognition you are filled with love so profound, that you know in every cell of your being, you will never ever let him go. And then, when the life story of your love keeps you apart for a while, you learn about the other, deeper, and invisible love bonds that tie and hold you together. And you understand that love has truly no limitations of time and space and that this long lost love of yours came from your very far past, most likely from another lifetime. And if it traveled and survived through death, surely a momentary separation is but a tiny flash in your tale of love everlasting. And always know, that each passing day without him, you are one day closer to seeing his beautiful eyes once again.

This Mudra will help you overcome grief of separation and nurture your heart.

Speak from Your Heart:

In our tale of love, conceived thru serendipity a
nd immaculate intervention from the Universe, I trust that we were
brought together with a higher purpose and every step on our journey is predestined, meaningful and clear.
Your momentary physical distance can not prevent your heart from beating with mine,
your whisper still buzzing in my ear, and your soft kiss melting on my skin.
Perhaps it is only with separation that we will understand how deep and everlasting our love is.
If it endured thru lifetimes with this kind of force, it is beyond indestructible.
And as I did before, I will wait for you forever, because that's how long our love shall reign.

Affirmation:
**I AM WITH YOU NOW,
THIS VERY MOMENT AND FOREVER.**

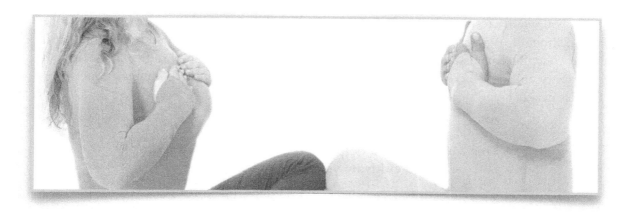

Sit with a straight back and face your partner, knees touching lightly. Lift up your hands and place them on your chest, palms facing the heart, all fingers together. Breathe and gaze into your partner's eyes and merge with him in the deepest way possible, with your mind, heart and soul. See yourself together in a most beautiful field of golden light, protected and nurtured, shielded from darkness and exalted in brightness of unconditional love. You are together no matter where you are, for physical distance is meaningless, what matters is the closeness of your two spirits, connected by ancient sacred bonds. Hold for three minutes. Open your heart while projecting unconditional love.

Breath:

Long, deep and slow.

Mudra for Inner Security

The love path that the two of you are walking on will show you many different views. There will be times when you will be passing nothing but endless fields of roses and the divine aroma lingering in the air will make everything seem most alluring. And when walking over the mountaintops, you will enjoy the magnificent expansion of your view, and marvel at the life secrets you'll discover together. But when you'll descend into the deep valleys where the sun sets early, and the evening chill envelops your back, this is when you will be tested. What will determine your resilience will be your own confidence in the strength of your love. If you resist the doubts of darkness to enter your mind and heart, you will remain solid side by side, together, conquering all and holding a clear vision of victory ahead. Everything in life is fleeting, but your love is everlasting and unending. Remember that, and never let go of each other's hand.

**This Mudra set will help you receive powerful insight
and cultivate your inner security**

Speak from Your Heart:

*When I open my heart to you and show you my sacred gems, I become more vulnerable,
and sometimes the cold draft of earthly mist clouds my inner compass of stability.
That is when my heart shivers at the thought of losing you,
and a coat of devastation descends upon my back.
I need you to remind me that you are here come rain or shine
and nothing will tear us apart, not even a final breath.
Then I will light up again and the fire in my heart will remain intact.*

Affirmation:
**WE ARE PROTECTED BY THE UNIVERSE
AND I AM WITH YOU ALWAYS.**

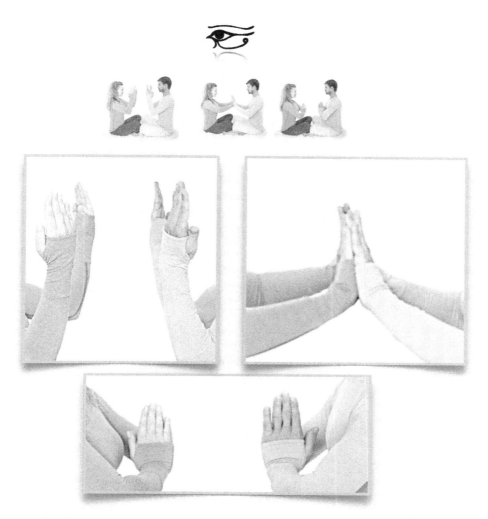

Sit with a straight back and face your partner, knees touching lightly. Lift up your hands, elbows to the side and elevated. Turn your palms towards you, all fingers together. Feel the healing energy from your hands envelop and strengthen you. Hold for three minutes. Now join your palms together with your partner's and lightly press them against each other. Hold and keep gazing into each other's eyes, feeling your energy blend and expand. Finally, end the set with the Mudra of divine worship, recognizing your everlasting connection to the Divine. The first Mudra activates your own power, the second magnifies joined forces of your love, and the third evokes the optimal protection when merging with the divine.Breathe and look kindly, gently and lovingly into your partner's eyes and project strength of love, and a sense of security to and for each other. See the divine being in your partner and envision brightness and light surrounding you in a protective shield. Practice for three minutes.

Breath:

Long, deep and slow.

Mudra for Confidence

Whatever happened to you in your life before your partner came across your path and changed the way the sun rises in the morning, all these past setbacks left an imprint on you. And because your past adventures may not have had a happy ending, you are inevitably unsure of your own self worth. Many of us search for shortcomings within ourselves and mistakenly believe even for a fleeting time, that it was all our own doing, our own fault, or our own imperfections that caused the failure of relationships past. However, reflect upon the situation from a distance and you will discover that it was precisely these experiences that brought you now to where you are, deserving, ready and capable to embrace and welcome the love meant and destined for your heart. So in fact you did not fail, but you ascended to prepare for the pinnacle of your heart's journey. You accomplished this and are now rewarded with the love of your life.

**This Mudra will imprint the vibration
of self-confidence in your mind and heart.**

Speak from Your Heart:
*I consciously leave the voices of my past behind and choose to listen to your song,
for your heart serenades with utmost beauty, never heard on earth before.
I choose to hear your words, the kindest ever spoken.
I choose to believe when you assure me to trust and jump off the cliff, because you will catch me in midair.
I choose to fall asleep in your arms carefree and open,
because I know tomorrow morning you will be here with me, blended in love.*

Affirmation:
**WE DESERVE THE GREATEST GIFTS
LIFE AND LOVE HAVE TO OFFER.**

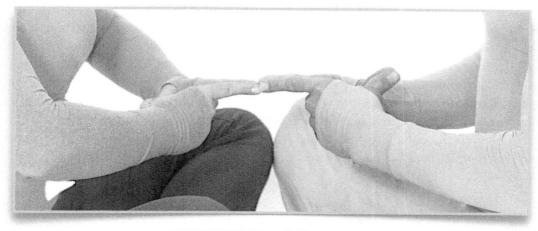

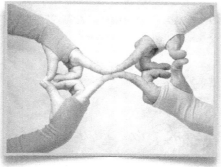

Sit with a straight back and face your partner, knees touching lightly. Lift the hands up to the solar plexus level and connect the index and thumb fingertips. The thumbs are pointing towards your solar plexus and the index fingers away from your body towards your partner. Bend the middle, ring and pinky fingers and place them back to back starting at the first knuckle. Notice how you've created a small heart with your fingers and palms. Now connect your connected index fingertips with those of your partner. Feel the powerful surge of energy run thru your both and transform the energy field within and all around you. Breathe and gaze into your partner's eyes and completely let go and open up to love and stillness. Project unconditional love into your partner's heart and envelop him with light and love. Practice for three minutes.

Breath:

Long, deep and slow.

Mudra for Finding Solutions

Life is supposed to be a puzzle, a learning journey, an adventure and an unpredictable experience. If we knew everything ahead of time, we could not grow in the same way. And even if it happens that you know certain things ahead of time, you don't know everything and all possible options that may follow as a consequence of your choices and decisions. So when the two of you come heads up against a challenge, remain steady and centered and don't allow emotions to take over, bringing up old fears that will decide for you. Together your unified wisdom has the ability to resolve anything, anytime and anyplace. Remember that forces joined are much fiercer than those of a single warrior.

So support your partner instead of fighting him, allow him to lead, and guide you thru the maze safely into the light. Trust and love his desire to be the leader, and remain the ever reliable partner, protect his back, guard him from all sides, always as a loyal ally with a heart of gold.

**This Mudra of wisdom will magnify your own ability
for foresight and higher understanding.**

Speak from Your Heart:

*I love being a team that we are, for in the spirit of togetherness
I know our alliance is etched deep within our souls and nothing can or will break this ancient bond.
When we are not sure how to proceed, I will remain calm and centered with you,
and help you stay the same, so that we can recognize the challenge
is not going to separate us, but unite us even deeper.
This will assure that our journey is guided by the best navigation system in existence -
the divine power itself.*

Affirmation:
**TOGETHER WE ARE WISE BEYOND THIS WORLD,
OUR DEVOTED LOVE IS GUIDING THE WAY.**

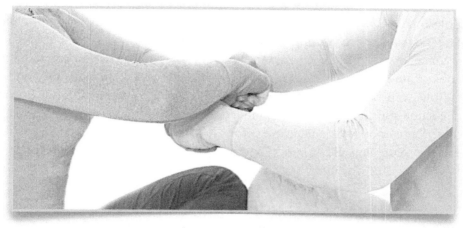

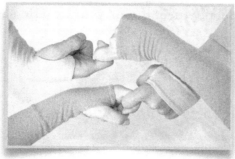

Sit with a straight back and face your partner, knees touching lightly. Lift the hands up to the solar plexus level and make fists with both hands, leaving the thumbs on the outside and index fingers stretched. Now hook your right index finger with right index finger of your partner. Your palm is facing down and his is facing him. Likewise hook your left index finger with his left index finger, your palm is facing you and his palm is facing down. Now gently pull and put pressure on these hooked index fingers, feeling a strong energy current between you, flowing through your hands, arms and body. Breathe and look deeply into each other's eyes and be conscious of the tremendous strength between you and the force that your unified action creates. Project unconditional love, loyalty, trust and confidence while gazing at each other. Practice for three minutes.

Breath:

Long, deep and slow.

Mudra for Recognizing Lessons

Sometimes when you walk through a most beautiful and mysterious forest, you come to a fork on the path. Should you follow the soft and mossy way deeper into the unknown wilderness, or pick the other, familiar and safe option? If your curiosity seduces you into a direction unknown yet inviting, you are open to anything. When after a while, deep darkness descends and you can't find your way back, you know you made the wrong turn. Yes, after a while you will be safe again, but most likely after quite an ordeal and a measure of fear. If next time while on the same path, you make the same turn on the road and get lost, you'll know even better this turn was wrong yet again. How many times do you need to repeat the same journey, before you understand and remember where to turn? If we walk together, this lesson won't take long, for we'll have each other and most likely will never repeat the same mistake again. Together, we can learn faster and accelerate our ascension.

**This Mudra set for guidance will help you find
the deeper meaning of your experiences.**

Speak from Your Heart:

*Discovering unknown worlds with you is my favorite adventure.
And while we may get lost, it never frightens me.
I know we will unravel the secrets and resolve the puzzle created and planted for us by the universe.
And if we fail at first, we will always take the responsibility together
and will never blame or fault each other.
And with time we'll become so in tune, that we'll see the lessons before they happen,
and our life's journey will flow smoothly like a beautiful weightless being,
sliding across the surface of a lake.
We'll learn together, overcome together and soar together high up to the sky.*

Affirmation:
**WE ASK THE DIVINE FOR DEEPER UNDERSTANDING,
WE ARE OPEN AND RECEPTIVE.**

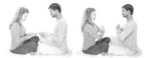

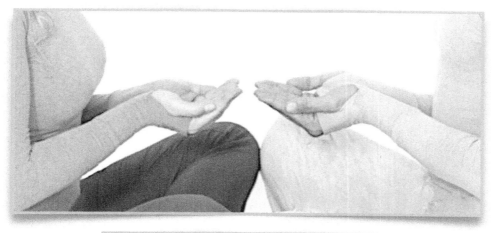

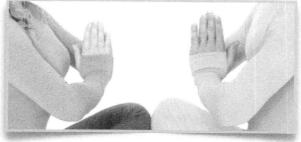

Sit with a straight back and face your partner, knees touching lightly. Lift the hands up to the solar plexus level and turn the palms up towards the sky. The sides of the hands with little fingers are touching, hands are held relaxed and slightly cupped. **Gaze into your hands**, relaxing your eyes, not focusing on a clear point, but expanding your vision to a level of higher energy sensory perception. See the universal light streaming into your cupped hands, bringing you gifts, answers and clarity about your challenges. Practice for three minutes. Be clear with your questions and take time to hear the answers. Now place your hands in front of your heart palm to palm, and hold the Mudra of divine worship for three minutes while gazing into your partner's eyes with love, devotion and compassion. Expand your heart and observe the divinity in your partner. Practice for three minutes.

Breath:

Long, deep and slow.

Part Six

Embellish Your Spirit

My soul has a voice, but it can only be heard in silence.
It has a language, but it can only be understood by someone who loves me.
It has a desire, but it can only be fulfilled with you.
I've been on my journey, completed assignments, but now that you're near,
I know that together, we can hold the light higher, shine brighter, be stronger.
I've missed you and our love, for we are meant to be together and never apart.
Yes, my soul is beautiful, but together with yours, they both blend into divine.

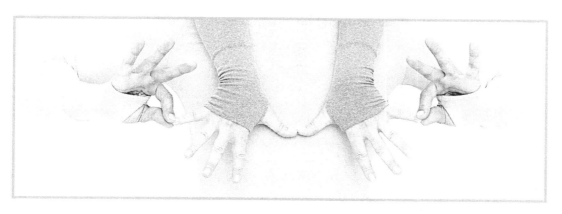

Mudra of Magnifying Your Soul Power

Mudra for Prosperity

While in this world, we all have to deal with one indisputable fact - the energy currency measured by money. For some it is easier than the others, but the riches of this world are all temporary and in no way a true measure of one's accomplishment or success. True prosperity is invisible, untouchable and of ethereal nature, unable to be measured by earthly law. Your soul's pure intention, your good deeds, your ability to love unconditionally - how can you put that on a scale and quote a number? Together as a team you need to be awakened and conscious of this unseen measuring system and never allow the earthly concept to get too close to your love. The heart does not measure prosperity with money, the heart does not understand this language, for it is the mind and ego that play that game. Your spiritual mindfulness and your ability to love unconditionally are your greatest wealth, immune to earthly measures and truly everlasting. This, you can't buy, but must earn through lifetimes of study, without cheating or avoidance, but through honest, raw and endless lessons.

**This Mudra will activate your ability to attract,
manifest and sustain prosperity in all realms**

Speak from Your Heart:

*To me, you are the most prosperous mate, for you can speak the language of my soul,
hear the song of my heart, understand the message in my eyes, and sense what I am dreaming of.
Somebody with worldly toys as distractions for their manipulation of power,
makes me cautious and estranged.
It is only a person of your spiritual stature that understands the wealth of my heart.
You, with your exceptional strength of character, unmatched attunement to my spirit,
and supreme ability to love and see me better than anyone ever did or will -
to me, you are wealthy beyond measure.*

Affirmation:
**THE UNIVERSE PROVIDES US
WITH EVERYTHING WE NEED OR WANT.**

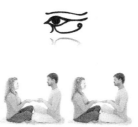

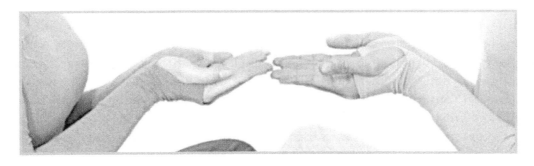

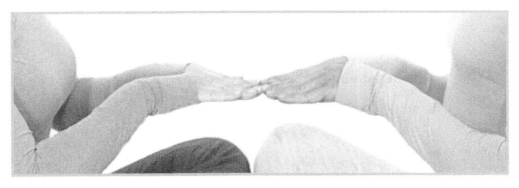

Sit with a straight back and face your partner, knees touching lightly. Lift the hands up to the solar plexus level and turn the palms up towards the sky. The sides of the hands with little fingers are touching, hands are held relaxed and slightly cupped. Now connect your fingertips lightly with your partner's. Turn the palms facing down and touch the index finger side of the hands together, thumbs slightly tucked away. Repeat the movement back to palms turned up towards the sky position. With each movement of changing your hands, you inhale and exhale in an even but comfortably fast paced tempo. Thru the practice your fingertips are lightly connected to your partner's. Breathe short, fast breath of fire. Look into your partner's eyes and remain steady with the breath and changing Mudra positions. See the divine wealth in your partner, the immeasurable richness of his soul, the immense love in his eyes and the overwhelming love of his heart enveloping you both. Project unconditional love to him with intention, open heart and every cell of your being. Know that together you are forever taken care of and provided for. Practice for three minutes.

Breath:

Short, fast breath of fire.

Mudra for Rediscovering Yourselves

It is human nature that we rush through life and rarely take a moment to be still, and truly soak up all the beauty that surrounds us. And yet, it is in the intricate detail of a flower's bloom where its spirit resides, hidden to all who can't see further, deeper and subtler. And it is a true marvel to see a flower open up towards the sun in the morning and stretch its petals with such speed you wonder who is inside, longing with such desire for sunlight. The love between two people is like a flower, it goes through seasons and changes constantly, sometimes within hours in a day. It's always longing for light and affection. When you and your lover graduate from the honeymoon phase and begin a new chapter, sometimes you may feel lost and confused, that's because you don't know how to navigate. This is the moment when you can rediscover each other, for you are ready to reach new levels of appreciation and transcend previous limitations. Nurture your love as you would a most delicate flower and it will bloom perpetually, expanding its petals and reaching for bliss.

**This Mudra set will help you alter and
expand the way you see and experience each other.**

Speak from Your Heart:

*And even if I know you deeply, there are still
those mysterious undiscovered corners of your heart that I long to unveil.
And in the depths of your soul, there is an endless oasis of such beauty, that I still need to explore.
And with each look that you give me, I see a new nuance
in your mesmerizing eyes that tells me there is more, an infinite world where you came from.
I want to travel there and explore the secret mysteries with you, feel the vastness of your soul
and hear the fine vibration of your being, resonating in accord with mine.
I will always journey on my favorite mission,
to follow you deeper into the endless ocean of love that you are.*

Affirmation:

**I SEE YOU... I LOVE YOU... I AM YOU...
AND YOU ARE ME.**

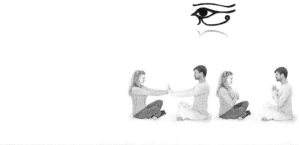

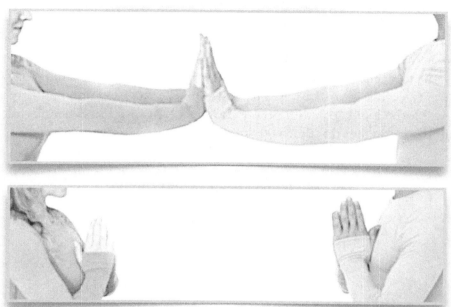

Sit with a straight back and face your partner, knees are not touching for you are a foot of distance apart. Lift the hands up to the heart level and stretch them towards each other, placing the palms together against each other. Apply gentle pressure and feel each other's energy through palms, hands, leading towards your heart and traveling through your entire being. See the divine in your partner and feel the magnified subtle energy power between you. Breathe and hold for three minutes. Now place the palms together in Mudra of Divine Worship. Gaze deeply into your partner's eyes and completely let go. Become one with him and drop all sense of limitations. Breathe and hold for three minutes. Now return to the first position and extend your arms to touch your partner's hands again - palm to palm. You will experience an interesting occurrence. Even though you did this Mudra in the beginning, this second time the Mudra will feel very different. Your ethereal energy body has expanded, reconnected and blended, and the joined merged energy body is offering an entirely different sense of your liaison. Breathe and hold for three minutes. Observe and enjoy another embodiment of your love, while projecting unconditional love and limitless affection towards your partner.

Breath:

Long, deep and slow.

Mudra for Equality

Through history we have battled each other over power and control. In our love, we need to break all barriers and ancient limitations that only suffocate our spirit and deprive our love of even ground. Recognizing the greatest value in each other instead of threat, opening our eyes to the beauty in each other instead of judgment, hearing the words of wisdom from different perspectives instead of competition… those are the qualities we must engage in our sphere of love. How can we cultivate that? Mudras will help you set up a perfectly balanced energetic base, so that you can climb up the ladder of love and maintain equality, each step of the way. The first step may feel awkward, but with each step higher you will ascend and soar with power combined, for instead of fighting each other, you will fight the world, but this time with love, the greatest weapon of them all.

**This Mudra will balance and equate
the energy and fortitude between you.**

Speak from Your Heart:

*When I wake up in the morning and you are there for me with love and soothing lips,
reminding me of the night before when we both cried tears of love,
I remember how lovely it is to be free and limitless in our love for one another.
If we would succumb to limitations of the world,
this would confuse our pure hearts and perplex our infinite souls,
for they know each other as completely equal parts of one entity.
And while we traveled thru endless lifetimes
before finding each other once more, we know what it means to be perfectly identical,
for we pledged equality to the universe as two corresponding parts
of one glorious essence, forever united with love.*

Affirmation:
**WE ARE TWO PERFECT HALVES
OF ONE GLORIOUS SOUL.**

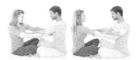

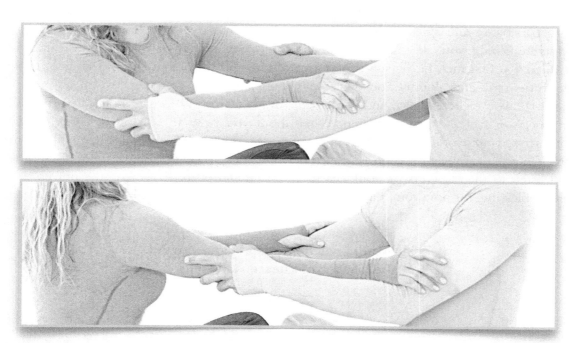

Sit with a straight back and face your partner, knees touching lightly. Lift the hands up and place them on the upper arms of your partner, just above the elbows. The woman holds her arms on the inside while the man places his hands on the outside of this position. Rest the hands on each other's upper arms into a comfortable position. Now inhale as you move back your right shoulder and move forward your left. Exhale when extending the right arm forward and moving back your left shoulder. Breathe in a comfortable long, deep and slow tempo, do not rush. While moving your shoulders, maintain a close and concentrated connection with your partner's eyes and observe the energy shifts within your physical, mental as well as emotional disposition. See his strength, power, determination but also his gentleness, consideration and compatibility with you. You will find a perfectly comfortable tempo that will suit you both and help you find balance through this Mudra. You will sense how together, you are indescribably stronger than alone. Project unconditional love and devotion to each other and your beautiful relationship. Practice for three minutes.

Breath:

Long, deep and slow.

Mudra for Maintaining Love

Because the sun shines every day, you forget how necessary it is. Because you see the blue sky right above you, you forget how essential it is. Because you pass the swaying trees each morning, you forget how extraordinary they are. Because you have seen roses before, you forget to pause and smell their divine scent. And because you see each other every day upon awakening, you take it for granted, and forget how much you wished and dreamed of it when you first met. If the sun is scarce in winter, you shiver and long for its rays. If the sky turns dark and gloomy, you dream of summer days. If the trees lose their leaves in chilly fall, you feel crestfallen and depressed. And if you never receive a delicate rose from anyone, you feel sad and forgotten. What about you two? If one of you was missing tomorrow, your world would crash and your eyes would cease shining. Remember how precious each and every second is, remember how lucky you are to have found each other and listen to the whispers of your heart. And each and every day, thank the universe for such a blessing, for now you finally belong.

**This Mudra will help sustain and expand
the love in your hearts and souls.**

Speak from Your Heart:

*Just because I can hear your voice when I need too, it doesn't mean that it ceased to warm my soul.
And when you speak the language of love, my heartstrings play a song so fine nobody can hear it but you.
And just because I can touch your hand and get lost in your embrace when I need you,
it doesn't mean that I don't want to return to you always and forever, for you are my true and only home.
And each time you kiss me, the world spins differently and a new galaxy is born.
You are always new to me, and I marvel at the endless shades of love in you.*

Affirmation:
**MY LOVE IS HERE FOR YOU,
ALWAYS AND FOREVER.**

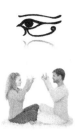

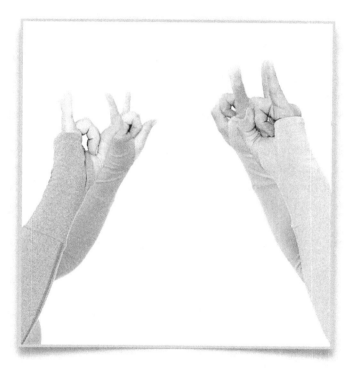

Sit with a straight back and face your partner, knees touching lightly. Lift the arms up so the elbows are at the shoulder level and lift the hands to the face level. Now stretch the index and little fingers, bend the middle and ring fingers, and cross the thumbs over the two bended middle fingers. Hold this position with the palms facing out, towards your partner. This is Mudra for Love. Breath is very specific of eight short inhalations and one long, deep exhale. With each set of short inhalations, feel your heart expanding and creating space for more love. Your ability for love is endless and everlasting. Look deeply into your partner's eyes and see the absolute divine power in him, permeate your combined auric space with unconditional love, devotion and gratitude that you have the gift of each other in your life. Feel the love in every cell of your being. Practice for three minutes.

Breath:

Eight short inhalations and one long, deep exhale.

Mudra for Establishing Compatibility

The sacred, secret combination of two people fitting perfectly is a wonder that can not be duplicated. There is so much more to it than it seems, and the complexities of energetic balance on a subtle level is what truly matters. A perfectly compatible relationship has less to do with similar interest or tastes, and more with a sacred component of two soul's uniquely synchronized frequency resonance, mutual ethereal attraction, sustainability of their equal awareness, and the rare gene of endurance thru parallel growth. When two people connect, their subtle energy sensors examine each other and instantaneously know if they are in harmony. This invisible meeting happens on ethereal realms, and when someone's energy is with you, hovering in your mind and heart, this compatibility test already occurred and spiritually you are already together, blended in a completely synchronized way. It is your individual state of evolution that plays a decisive role in optimal compatibility, one that surpasses all earthly obstacles and overcomes all society's differences. Trust the universe when it puts you two together, and consciously open your heart so that when destiny sends you true love, you await with recognition and receptivity.

**This Mudra set will expand your ethereal space and
establish a field for perfect interaction.**

Speak from Your Heart:

*When you go through your life without meeting a person that understands you
in the deepest corners of your soul, you expect that perhaps they do not exist.
And yet your heart keeps hoping that when your love appears, you will recognize them once again. I
recognize the divine gifts in my life and you are such a destined inevitability for me.
And when you understand and feel me so profoundly as you do,
for me all questions are answered and all doubts are erased in an instant.
Please do not disbelieve this sacred gift upon us, for in my heart I know,
we are what we longed for, for so long.*

Affirmation:
**THIS IS OUR SACRED SPACE
OF MAJESTIC POWER AND LOVE.**

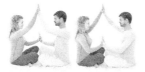

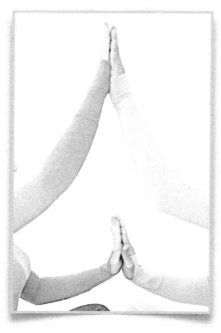
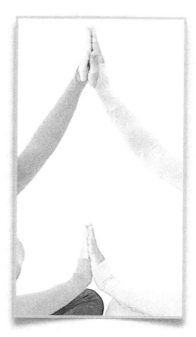

Sit with a straight back and face your partner, knees touching lightly. Lift the hands up to the heart area and turn the palms facing out, towards your partner. Connect your palms with your partner's and be aware of the tremendous energy current that flows thru your hands and merges your ethereal bodies. Now begin the practice by inhaling and extending your right hand (your partner's left) up high, so that the elbows are stretched completely. When you exhale bring the right hand down and lift up the left hand (your partner's right) and repeat the same motion on that side. The inhalation is always when you lift the right hand, exhalation when you lift the left.

For your partner it is the opposite. Practice for three minutes. Breathe long, deep and slow with each motion of the hand. Now reverse the pattern, inhaling while extending your left arm (your partner's right) and exhaling while lifting your right hand (your partner's left). Look into his eyes with love and complete inner peace, opening your mind and heart to absorb his essence and flow with his energy. Together you are synchronizing your frequency so that it resonates at the optimal compatible and harmonious level. Project divine love and acceptance. Practice for three minutes.

Breath:

Breathe long, deep and slow with each motion of the hands.

Mudra for Magnifying Respect

Like with everything else in your life, it is you as an individual who sets parameters, boundaries and limitations on how you allow others to treat you. It is an instant reflection of how you treat yourself. Hopefully you have had time to reflect and work upon this trait so that when you'll meet your true love, you can begin your love journey from a beautiful point. In such a case you will attract a compatible and harmonious lover who will respect you as you desire. If you begin your love journey together with a lack of self respect, this will require tending to and your conscious effort to understand, take responsibility for, and improve this dynamic. If the two of you started on great footing, but have with time and certain events noticed that your mutual respect has faded and diminished, you need to work on this together and repair the damage, just as you would fix the wings on your glider. It will take both of you to mend the tear, if you want to avoid a crash. But just think how breathtaking your view will be, sailing above the clouds.

This Mudra of concentration will help you eliminate self - doubt and nurture mutual respect.

Speak from Your Heart:

When I get so close to you, I know you see all my imperfections and faults.
This isn't easy for me, even though I have nothing to hide.
I have peace about all decisions and past actions in my life, as I always respected myself.
And yes, the worldly price seemed high, but the spiritual reward was higher.
And no matter what you say or feel about yourself in a moment of self-doubt,
I do and will always respect you, because I recognize the magnitude and brilliance of your soul -
beyond magnificent and oh, so pure.

Affirmation:
**WE LOVE, RESPECT AND APPRECIATE EACH OTHER
TODAY AND FOREVER.**

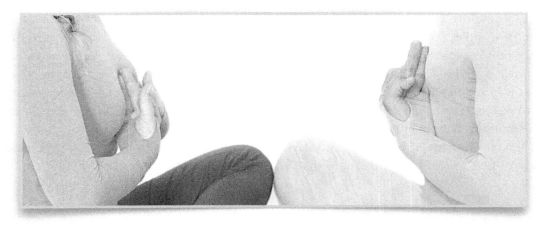

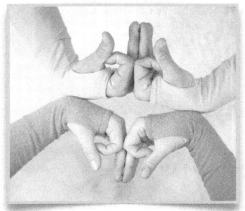

Sit with a straight back and face your partner, knees touching lightly. Lift the hands up to the heart level and place them lightly on your chest. Now curl the index fingers into your thumbs, and connect them at the index knuckles back to back. Keep all other fingers straight and place them back to back across the entire length of them. Breathe long, deep and slow. Look into your partner's eyes and project unconditional love, seeing divine in him. See the beauty of his soul, understand the treasure of his love, see yourself in a loving and kind way and project this vibration onto him. Practice for three minutes.

Breath:

Long, deep and slow.

Mudra for Tenderness

When you first meet, the emotions aroused and desires awakened propel you into a state of utter bliss and hypnotic fever. All you want is to be near each other and swim in this amazing bubble of love and passion. You instantaneously know how to be tender, sweet, loving, and adore your lover like the world is ending tomorrow and these are your final hours. With time, your passion has to adjust just like a match when you light it, the first combustion is explosive, and then it's up to you how long you can sustain the flame. When your love is multidimensional and not just purely based on a physical adventure, when your souls are intertwined and merged on the highest level, your flame never goes out, in fact it takes over in a ceaseless flare. What makes a difference in the experience and quality of this bond, is your ability to at anytime and anyplace instantaneously offer your lover the most tender moment of adoration and devotion. With that you can drown any argument, outburst of fear or ego. If you can do that, you have mastered the art of love.

**This Mudra set will help you develop,
embellish and deepen your tender devotion to each other.**

Speak from Your Heart:

*If you would hold my heart in your hands, you would feel its vulnerable flutter.
You would understand how all it needs and wants is your tender love, your gentle,
soft caress and the protective haven of your care. No matter what I say or do
in a weak moment of fear, do not forget that underneath it all,
my heart is always like that, sometimes hiding in pride,
dressed in fear, or overshadowed by ego.
My heart remains and continues to beat for the one and only that I love.
It longs for your affection and warmth, because it needs it like air to survive and live on.
Please my love, be tender with me, for I will always be most gently delicate with you as well.*

Affirmation:

**THE PASSAGE TO MY HEART IS OPEN FOR YOU,
I AM YOURS.**

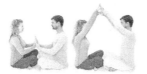

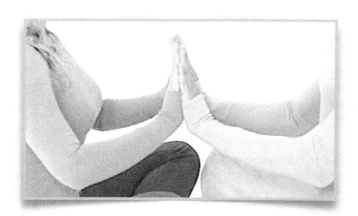

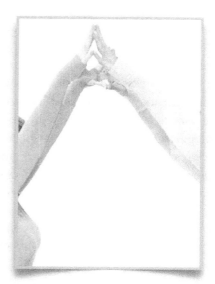

Sit with a straight back and face your partner, knees touching lightly. Lift the hands up to the level of your heart and hold the palms facing away from your body, towards your partner. All the fingers are held together. Now touch your partner's palms with yours and apply gentle pressure. Inhale and lift your connected palms up towards the sky, while spreading the fingers apart and **connecting only with fingertips**. All fingers are stretched and the pressure you feel between each other's fingers creates a strong energy flow. Now exhale and bring the hands back to the original position and again connect the fingers and full palms together. Repeat the motion each time with inhalation rising your hands above your head, only fingertips touching, and exhaling when descending hands, connecting entire palms.

Breath is long, deep and slow with each motion of the hands. Gaze into your partner's eyes, projecting love and openness of your heart. Each time you elevate your hands, connect with the image of a passage you are building for your emotions of love, kindness, gentleness and tender thoughts for each other. Practice for three minutes.

Breath:

Breathe long, deep and slow with each motion of the hands.

Mudra for Releasing Expectations

We all have days or even months, when for no particular reason, we feel out of sorts. And you may believe that it is your partner who disappointed you, so you blame him, mope around and wait. It's like when you think that by dressing up, you will see a new, beautiful version of yourself, so you find a most exquisite dress, but when you put it on and gaze upon your reflection, you don't like what you see. The dress that looked like a dream, now looks drab. Do you think it is really the dress that's amiss, or is it possible you simply don't like yourself? Similarly in a relationship, you have certain expectations of how everything will be rosy, easy and done for you. Well, it won't. Even if you pressure your partner to create that magical fairy tale scenario, you won't be able to live in it, because you can't find that fairy tale within. So be truly honest with yourself when placing high expectations upon your partner. He is not the answer to your happiness, you are. Once you accept that, the burden will be off his shoulders and together you can breathe a sigh of relief. And you, lighten up and learn to appreciate little things, for it is not the size of the lake, but the purity of the water in it that matters.

**This Mudra for releasing worries
will diminish your restlessness and set you free.**

Speak from Your Heart:

*Truthfully, I expected too much of myself and when I couldn't measure up,
I transferred that expectation to other places
when in fact expectation was just a cranky, pestering habit of my ego.
So I locked it up and threw away the key, and now I can finally enjoy myself
without the scolding voice and nagging whispers.
Now it's just you and I, free and open like two seagulls in the sky,
flying with the wind, expecting and knowing we'll remain in the air, effortlessly so.
And yes, I hope we'll be happy and in love forever, and I know you wish the same.
But we'll release all expectations, for we both know we have nothing to worry about.
It's all here.*

Affirmation:

**WE RELEASE ALL EXPECTATIONS
AND ALLOW THE UNIVERSE TO GUIDE OUR WAY**

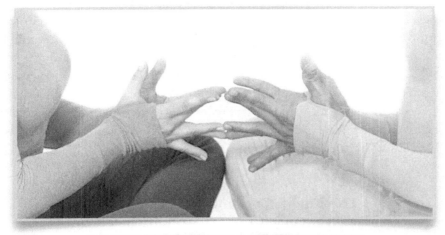

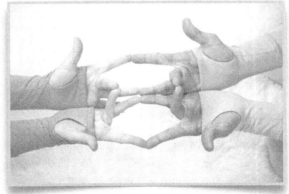

Sit with a straight back and face your partner, knees touching lightly. Lift the hands up to the level of solar plexus and turn the open palms up, towards the sky. Now place the open palms next to each other, little fingers touching along the outside line. Connect the fingertips of your middle fingers, point them up towards the sky, and extend all other fingers. Now bring the hands closer with your partner's and connect the tips of your index and ring fingers with his, creating a beautiful Mudra for releasing worry. Thumbs are pointing up towards the sky, little fingers towards the ground. Breathe long, deep and slow. Gaze into your partner's eyes and see the pure love in his being. See yourself in his eyes and blend into oneness. Breathe and practice for three minutes.

Breath:

Long, deep and slow.

Mudra for Learning Silence

Yes, some of us are talkers and love to chirp endlessly like birds on a springtime morning. And apparently, we expect our partner to be like us. And they may listen to you and for a while with honest interest, but when you repeat another version of the same story for the third time, they will get bored and forget to hide it well. This should not become a reason for discontent, for you should strive to find a middle way, and learn to listen to the silence within you. Once you discover that magic, your sensing ability will expand to perceive the slightest change in your partner's mood. And very discreetly, two more characters will appear, named harmony and peace, and the three of them together will surround you two with such a fine shield of protection, you will feel like you are floating in another world. You and your love in complete silence, and how divine the soothing sound of his balmy sigh on your neck, just because he loves you so.

**This Mudra for calming will help you
distance yourself from all worldly chatter.**

Speak from Your Heart:

*I love conversing with you and hearing your views on life and all it entails.
But I also love the silence we can hold, the stillness when we know nothing else is needed,
because the two of us are enough.
This for me is complete profound peace, a sense of letting go of all the armors,
shields and covers, and just enjoying the experience of being.
The unspoken language of silence has a vocabulary so advanced, no words can match its bounty.
Now we speak with our minds and most of all, with the pureness of our hearts.
This is flawless, this is love.*

Affirmation:

**IN STILLNESS OF THIS MOMENT
OUR SOULS MERGE IN ONE.**

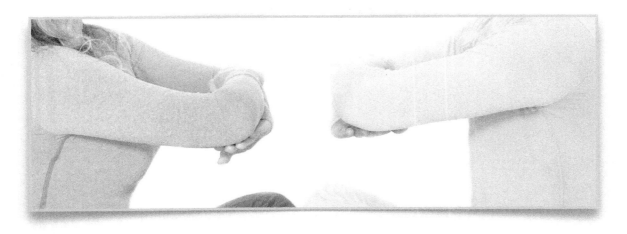

Sit with a straight back and face your partner, knees touching lightly. Lift the hands up to heart level and bend your elbows. Place the right hand on your left, palms facing down, right hand resting on the forearm of your left forearm. Your partner should practice this Mudra by mirroring your hand positions - left arm resting on the right forearm. Fingers are together, palms facing down. The woman is calming her mind, while the man is calming the emotional side of his nature. This way, they meet in a neutral place in-between, and establish an ideal place of silent communication. Breathe long, deep and slow. Look into your partner's eyes and project love, completely let go, as if melting into each other's depth within. Open up your perception of mastering silent communication, project love, peace and harmony and remain utterly serene. Practice for three minutes.

Breath:

Long, deep and slow.

Part Seven

Soul Mate & Twin Flame Ascension

I know you see me as my true Spirit entity.
I feel you in my heart and soul, we are connected eternally, part of each other's essence, forever bound by ancient love.
Our journey has brought us back together after many incarnations of distance in time and space.
But our love remained, untouched, untarnished, everlasting,
it grew so much stronger and now,
we are untouchable.
The only touch that exists is the one between us.

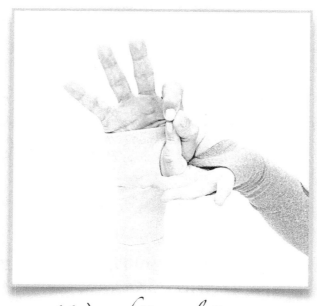

Mudra of Eternal Creation

Mudra for Trusting Unconditional Love

Unconditional love is like a most ethereal otherworldly butterfly. It takes a long time in gestation, a deep profoundly transformative process is taking place while the being exists in many different versions, all not incredibly appealing. And after this long and formidable journey, on a predestined day, a miracle happens and a most glorious astounding being appears, far superior than its previous incarnations, not only in its beauty and appeal, but in its ability to fly. Free at last. Similarly, you travel through many life journeys before you earn the ability to truly love unconditionally. It requires a pure and open heart, immaculate intention for selfless service to the world, and endless patience to wait while others learn. Your road may be especially lonely at times, and when you lastly meet your match, recognition will be instantaneous and your wings will open up for your final flight into ascension. Trust and know it is already in the making.

This Mudra will help you trust to open your hearts
and raise your pure emotions into ascension.

Speak from Your Heart:

I opened my heart without restrictions and allowed you to enter and touch every string of my inner harp.
And because you know how to play my sacred melody, I can sing along, ever so gently.
This breathtaking duet can only happen with you and I.
And if I would want to lock you up in the lush chambers of my heart,
you would feel frightened and wonder why I don't trust you, because you trust me.
So my heart remains open, you may fly away to feel the courage in your wings and the freedom of your soul.
I love you without conditions and in my heart I know you will always return, because our sacred melody
keeps us alive.

Affirmation:
MY LOVE FOR YOU IS DIVINELY LIMITLESS
AND PURE.

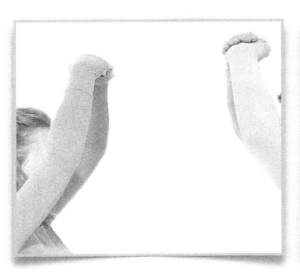 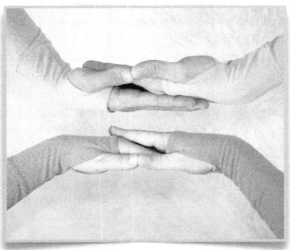

Sit with a straight back and face your partner, knees touching lightly. Begin by lifting your hands up above your head. Place the right hand on top of the left, palms facing down, thumb tips touching and lightly pressed together. *If men practice this Mudra alone, the left palm is on top of the right.*

Breath is short, fast, breath of fire. Practice for three minutes. Completely let go of any thoughts and merge into your partner's eyes, fearlessly and completely with an open heart and most generous feelings of love you can imagine. Know that between you there is only an indescribable feeling of love for nothing else exists, no fears, no expectations, no restless emotions and no time, there is only the two of you blended into one.

Breath:

Short, fast, breath of fire.

Mudra for Understanding Change

In this world of illusions and secret veils hiding other dimensions, we are tested and taught each and every day. Some days seem to be uneventful and others turn into a drama. But no two days are precisely identical, for no two seconds are. Everything is continuously spinning like the earth around the sun, and yet all we see is the sun rising or descending. We are in perpetual motion but crave stability. How can you be still when everything around you is spinning? You flow with it, like you learn to swim with the ocean's currents and not against them. As you two travel through life, know and accept that change is always present. And your love will also change, but do not fear, instead, open up to the possibility that it could be even more majestic than the day before. It is all in your ability to expand your perception. And trust me, when you leave this world, you won't lose each other, for your love is the most stable essence in your life, and when everything else ceases to exist, your love will live on. It may change its expression, but will live on eternally in the beyond.

**This Mudra of change will help you open up
and embrace new paths in your life.**

Speak from Your Heart:

*When I first heard your voice, my heart skipped a beat because I recognized you.
When I first saw your face, I saw our future and knew why you appeared.
You changed my perspective of time and space, for I felt you not near me, but inside my being.
Was this frightening? No, it was beautiful, because change brings you the most precious gifts of life.
And I know this is just the beginning, for trust me, I will change your world, and you have already changed mine.*

Affirmation:
**WITH EACH PASSING MOMENT
OUR LOVE GROWS DEEPER.**

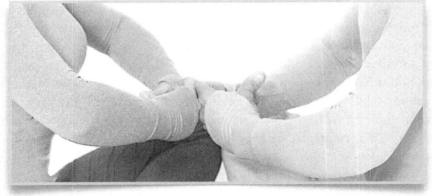

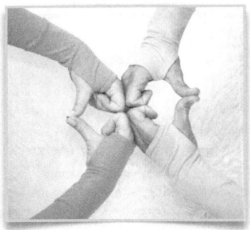

Sit with a straight back and face your partner, knees touching lightly. Lift the hands up, to the solar plexus level and bring your hands together. Curl your fingers into your palms leaving thumbs on the outside. Connect the thumb fingertips and point them towards your solar plexus. The knuckles of your bent fingers are touching. Now connect the backs of your hands with your partner's. Hold this Mudra of change, gently leaning against each other. **Breathe long, deep and slow.** Look deeply into each other's eyes and maintain eye contact while sending unconditional love towards each other's hearts. Relax into the Mudra and allow energy currents to interact and magnify your joined powers. Practice for three minutes.

Breath:

Long, deep and slow.

Mudra for Welcoming New Dynamics

When two souls that love each other with pure and open hearts, evolve and gain the ability to love unconditionally, they ascend to a higher realm. There, love is so much more than four letters, it is so much more than finding compatibility in earthly matters, it is much more than living together and enjoying a great life, it is so much more than having a family, it is so much more than watching the years go by. There is nothing wrong with that, but this is just a stop-over and not your final destination. When you are ready, the gates will open for you to enter a new world of higher love. Sometimes this happens after many years together, and other times upon meeting each other, you instantly initiate a profoundly cataclysmic energy shift that sets off an almost programmed capacity for spiritual ascension. When the two of you experience pure unity of two souls and understand the sacred and secret rule for entering celestial dimensions, the limited world as you know it, simply disappears. Allow yourself to be surprised and open up to the possibility, that there is much more to life than you ever possibly believed or imagined.

**This Mudra will prepare you for your conscious journey
to higher expressions of love.**

Speak from Your Heart:

*I know who you are to me, and you know who I am to you.
And while the world seems to spin in its usual way,
we know that there is another world within our souls
that expands beyond our ability to perceive.
And it is much grander that we both dare to dream.
When our love ascends, it will take us to where there is no sadness or sorrow,
no lacking or missing, there is just oneness and pure bliss.
I have waited for you, as you waited for me and the moment has come.*

Affirmation:

**WE ARE READY TO TRAVEL FURTHER, HIGHER,
TO OUR TRUE HOME.**

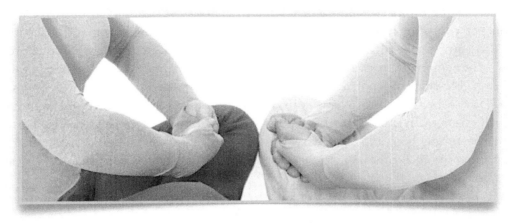

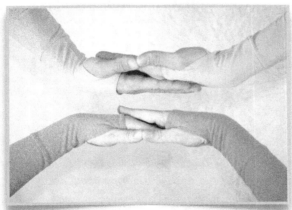

Sit with a straight back and face your partner, knees touching lightly. Place the hands in your lap, just slightly lifted. Both palms are turned up towards the sky. Now place the right hand below the left, resting. Thumb tips are connected, all fingers are stretched. **Breathe long, deep and slow.** Gaze into each other's eyes and establish an utter sense of calmness and peace. Project unconditional love to each other and hold a very clear focus, maintaining an open heart. Hold for three minutes.

Breath:

Long, deep and slow.

Mudra for Understanding Karmic Promises

Karma can be your greatest protector in time of need, and savior in times of desperation and sorrow. You created your karma, so it is your doing, and giving, and taking that is just bouncing back at you through different manifestations. Karma will bring you the rewards owed, open sacred doors of safe passage to hurl you out of a battlefield unharmed, it will help you get your "lucky break" and succeed seemingly overnight, when in fact it took lifetimes to earn it. But most importantly, it will suddenly present you with your greatest gift ever - your soulmate or twin flame. At that moment of great fortune, remember, this is your karmic blessing and not a debt. This ultimate reward brings with it a few sacred mysteries, yet to be unlocked by you both. Karmic promises are made before we are born and remain your main mission to be accomplished during your earthly travels. This final assignment can only be completed by two equal souls that are unconditionally prepared to risk everything for each other. Once they do, their souls are evermore free and their earthly karma is finalized.

**This Mudra of two wings will help you understand
and master your final karmic assignment.**

Speak from Your Heart:

*We have known each other for millenniums through heaven and hell,
thru battles and victories, thru life and death,
and we always found our way back to each other.
I have missed you so, that I almost forgot how it is when we are One.
But now that we are here once more, I will fulfill my promise
and give you my heart and soul so we can ascend to our true home.
Do not fear, you won't ever lose me again, I am here now, and this is our final dance on earth.
Let's make it an unforgettably victorious one.*

Affirmation:
WE ARE REUNITED AND ON OUR WAY HOME.

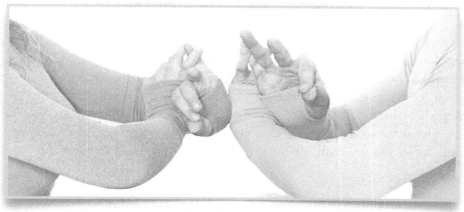

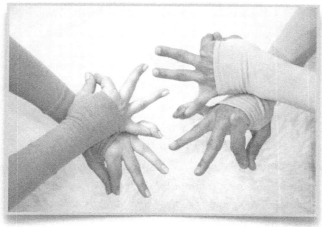

Sit with a straight back and face your partner, knees touching lightly. Place the hands in front of your heart, elbows comfortably below shoulder level. Turn the palms outwards toward your partner, and connect your index fingers with thumbs, all other fingers are apart and stretched. Now cross the right hand over left and hook your little fingers with each other, pulling them apart gently. Hold steady and do not lower your arms. Look lovingly into your partner's eyes and reveal the deepest emotions from the hidden corners of your heart. Open up your energy field and merge your love with his, while feeling strong energy currents flow from your open palms. Project unconditional love and trust. Hold for three minutes.

Breath:

Long, deep and slow.

Mudra for an Unbreakable Bond

When you love someone, you see everything through a very sensitive lens of your heart's vulnerability. You are in the world of adoration and your energy field is merged with that of your lover. This is a special sphere where you experience otherworldly beauty and spellbinding passion, all things lovely yet out of your control. When another, perhaps unknown or negative element enters your sacred space, your first reaction will be fear. You don't want to lose the balmy safety of this cocoon you created and everything appears like a predator. However, even if a challenging experience sends you thru a whirlwind of turmoil, it is up to you to overcome and defeat this adversary. And you will both emerge stronger and only thru this process, slowly but surely, you become truly unconquerable. And finally, you can be grateful for every obstacle that ever came your way, because it helped you test, reinforce, and secure the unbreakable bond that you now hold.

**This Mudra of powerful energy will solidify
and protect your ethereal bond.**

Speak from Your Heart:

*I know in my far distant memory that we have loved and lost each other many times.
The destiny tore us apart and yet it brought us together again,
giving in to our soul's longing and unbreakable force.
So we conquered death and pledged to find each other no matter what obstacles of time and space.
And you see, we cheated death again for it is powerless against us,
and now it's too late to pull us apart for we are no longer two people,
but two flames forever residing in one majestic soul.*

Affirmation:

**WE ARE ETERNALLY BOUND BY OUR PLEDGE
OF UNCONDITIONAL LOVE FOR EACH OTHER.**

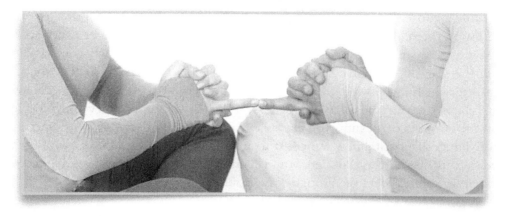

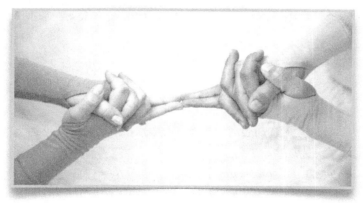

Sit with a straight back and face your partner, knees touching lightly. Lift the hands up to your solar plexus area, and interlace the fingers. Woman places the right thumb on top of her left, and the man places his left thumb on top of his right thumb. Extend the ring fingers and stretch them completely, touching along the insides. Now connect the ring fingertips with your partner's and feel the powerful energy current surge through your fingers. Gaze into your partner's eyes and project unconditional love and trust in your empowering connection and devotion to each other. Remain centered and focused, and observe the change in energy dynamics between your two energy bodies, interlacing and merging into one.Hold for three minutes.

Breath:

Long, deep and slow.

Mudra for Synchronizing Your Future

We all have dreams about our life and sometimes we are very good at pursuing them. Other times we forget them, and allow life to toss us around like a helpless shell of a ship in a stormy sea. When you learn to hold on to your dreams and visions of your future, you become a conscious participant in your life. Your lover has his own dreams and most likely a lot of them are quite harmonious with yours. But when you are very set in your mind how certain things should and must happen in order to reach your dreams, you stand in the way of the universe helping you. Certainly we can admit that the universe with its overwhelming power drives events with a certain cosmically aligned navigation system, which you can't possibly compete with. When you stop intervening and learn to fly with the currents of destiny, you create a synchronicity with the universe and enter the zone of limitless possibilities. When you and your lover allow your own dreams to interweave with the universal design, you will enter the space of complete alignment. And that's what we call the state of ultimate synchronicity.

This Mudra for better perception will help open your ability to recognize future opportunities.

Speak from Your Heart:

I know you have your dreams and I have mine. But in that hazy vision of our approaching future,
I always see you alongside me, your beautiful eyes following mine,
and your lips whispering reassuring words of love.
I realize that we are in this dream now and suddenly time and surroundings cease to exist.
My dream becomes you and I, and the whole galaxy is in alignment with our love.
Could it be that nothing else matters but us, and we are fortunate to be living our dreams here and now?
If the past, present and future are all fictional, I am content in this timeless existence with you.

Affirmation:
WE TRUST THE UNIVERSE
TO HELP US FULFILL OUR DREAMS.

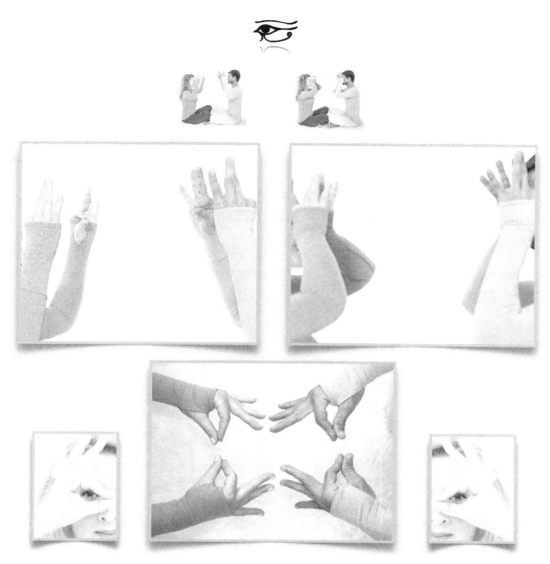

Sit with a straight back and face your partner, knees touching lightly. Connect your thumb and index fingers and stretch out the rest of the fingers. Now lift your arms up, elbows at shoulder level, and hold your arms to the sides. Inhale, long, deep and slow, while looking into your partner's eyes and slowly exhale while moving hands in front of your eyes. Look thru the circle openings in your hands and gaze at your partner with complete stillness and peace. Now inhale again and open up to move your hands into original position. This Mudra of adapting your perception helps you expand your inner vision and understand true elements of importance in your life. Project unconditional love and be open to insight, so you can understand and accept variations of your path to fulfillment of your dreams. Trust that the road the universe will present you with, will be far superior to your own plan. Practice for three minutes.

Breath:

Long, deep and slow.

Mudra for Recognizing Higher Purpose

When you know in your heart that you have found your perfect equal mate, your universe starts working under entirely different principles. It's like the earth's gravitation doesn't affect you, the time doesn't chase you, and the worldly desires evaporate. You understand that the ability to love unconditionally is the primary and most important aspect of your earthly experience. And this merging of two souls, this incredible magnified power establishes a new energy path of such magnitude that you realize with indisputable clarity, there is a much higher purpose at hand. And you know that together the two of you can actually establish an indestructible ray of light to shine upon all who are near. Your devotion to higher cause elevates you into realms of synchronized fluidity and opportunities manifest to share this light with others in a most loving, giving and healing way. Now you outgrow your personal desires and ascend into Light. You are home.

**This Mudra set will help you achieve
a higher state of merged consciousness.**

Speak from Your Heart:

*Yes, I have my dreams but they are always with you at my side.
My loyal partner that I trust with my most precious possessions - my heart and soul.
I rejoice in our purpose as messengers of light, the invincible ones, to fulfill our mission and conquer
all sorrow, bring light and joy to all who desire and pray for it.
I recognize my strength is complete with you at my side,
and when working together I feel absolute bliss and peace for
I know I am precisely where I am supposed to be -
working for the highest good with my best ally, friend and divine lover at my side.
Now, we are indestructible.*

Affirmation:
**WE MERGE OUR SPIRITS
TO UNITE AND ENLIGHTEN.**

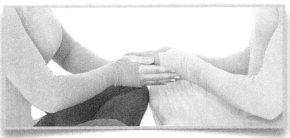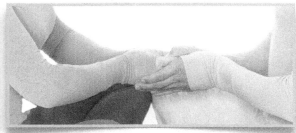

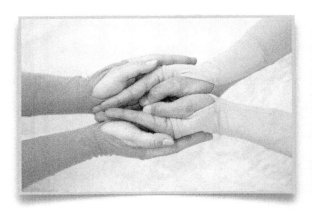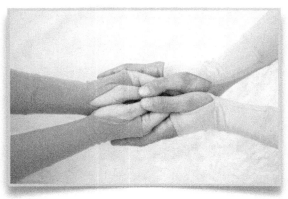

Sit with a straight spine. Lift your hands to solar plexus level and bring your palms together as if in a prayer pose. Bend the thumbs so they touch the fleshy mounds below the fingers of the same hand. Allow your partner to envelop your hands in his and finally, he will cover your thumbs with his. Hold for three minutes and then reverse the position, you holding his hands in yours. Again, hold for three minutes. Gaze into each other's eyes, deeply and with devotion, surrender and trust. When he holds your hands in his, allow him to radiate protective and loving energy into you, so that you may let go completely. When you change the position and hold his hands in yours, project utmost devotion and unconditional love, assuring him of your eternal presence and everlasting love. Now, you can tap into higher understanding of your joint bigger purpose.

Breath:

Long, deep and slow.

ABOUT THE AUTHOR

SABRINA MESKO   Ph.D.H. is a recognized Mudra authority and International and Los Angeles Times bestselling author of the timeless classic *Healing Mudras - Yoga for your Hands* translated into fourteen languages. She authored over twenty books on Mudras, Mudra Therapy, Mudras and Astrology, and meditation techniques.

Sabrina was born in Europe where she became a classical ballerina at an early age. In her teens she moved to New York and became a principal Broadway dancer and singer who turned to yoga to heal a back injury. Easter-trained but Western-based, she completed a several-year intensive study of teachings with world renowned Masters, one of whom entrusted her with bringing the sacred Mudra techniques to the West. She is a Yoga College of India certified Yoga Therapist.

Sabrina holds a Bachelors Degree in Sensory Approaches to Healing, a Masters in Holistic Science, and a Doctorate in Ancient and Modern Approaches to Healing from the American Institute of Holistic Theology. She is board certified from the American Alternative medical Association and American Holistic Health Association.

She has been featured in media outlets such as The Los Angeles Times, CNBC News, Cosmopolitan, the cover of London Times Lifestyle, The Discovery Channel documentary on Hands, W magazine, First for Women, Health, Web- MD, Daily News, Focus, Yoga Journal, Australian Women's weekly, Blend, Daily Breeze, New Age, the Roseanne Show and various international live television programs. Her articles have been published in world-wide publications. She hosted her own weekly TV show educating about health, well-being and complementary medicine. She is an executive member of the World Yoga Council and has led numerous international Yoga Therapy educational programs. She directed and produced her interactive double DVD titled *Chakra Mudras* - a Visionary awards finalist. Sabrina also created award winning international Spa and Wellness Centers and is a motivational keynote conference speaker addressing large audiences all over the world. Sabrina recently launched Arnica Press, a boutique Book Publishing House. Her mission is to discover, mentor, nurture and publish unique authors with a meaningful message, that may otherwise not have an opportunity to be heard.

She is the founder of MUDRA MASTERY ™ the world's only online Mudra Teacher and Mudra Therapy Education, Certification, and Mentorship program, with her certified graduates and therapists spreading these ancient teachings in over 26 countries around the world.

WWW.SABRINAMESKO.COM

Made in the USA
Las Vegas, NV
26 August 2022